Imaging of the Postoperative Spine

Editor

A. ORLANDO ORTIZ

NEUROIMAGING CLINICS OF NORTH AMERICA

www.neuroimaging.theclinics.com

Consulting Editor
SURESH K. MUKHERJI

May 2014 • Volume 24 • Number 2

ELSEVIER

1600 John F. Kennedy Boulevard • Suite 1800 • Philadelphia, Pennsylvania, 19103-2899

http://www.neuroimaging.theclinics.com

NEUROIMAGING CLINICS OF NORTH AMERICA Volume 24, Number 2
May 2014 ISSN 1052-5149, ISBN 13: 978-0-323-29717-2

Editor: John Vassallo (j.vassallo@elsevier.com)
Developmental Editor: Donald Mumford

Neuroimaging Clinics of North America (ISSN 1052-5149) is published quarterly by Elsevier Inc., 360 Park Avenue South, New York, NY 10010-1710. Months of issue are February, May, August, and November. Business and editorial offices: 1600 John F. Kennedy Blvd., Suite 1800, Philadelphia, PA 19103-2899. Business and editorial offices: 6277 Sea Harbor Drive, Orlando, FL 32887-4800. Periodicals postage paid at New York, NY, and additional mailing offices. Subscription prices are USD 360 per year for US individuals, USD 514 per year for US institutions, USD 180 per year for US students and residents, USD 415 per year for Canadian individuals, USD 655 per year for Canadian institutions, USD 525 per year for international individuals, USD 655 per year for international institutions and USD 260 per year for Canadian and foreign students and residents. To receive student/resident rate, orders must be accompanied by name of affiliated institution, date of term, and the *signature* of program/residency coordinator on institution letterhead. Orders will be billed at individual rate until proof of status is received. Foreign air speed delivery is included in all *Clinics* subscription prices. All prices are subject to change without notice. POSTMASTER: Send address changes to *Neuroimaging Clinics of North America*, Elsevier Health Sciences Division, Subscription Customer Service, 3251 Riverport Lane, Maryland Heights, MO 63043. Telephone: 1-800-654-2452 (U.S. and Canada); 314-447-8871 (outside U.S. and Canada). Fax: 314-447-8029. E-mail: journalscustomerservice-usa@elsevier.com (for print support); journalsonlinesupport-usa@elsevier.com (for online support).

Reprints. For copies of 100 or more of articles in this publication, please contact the Commercial Reprints Department, Elsevier Inc., 360 Park Avenue South, New York, NY 10010-1710. Tel.: 212-633-3874; Fax: 212-633-3820; E-mail: reprints@elsevier.com.

Neuroimaging Clinics of North America is covered by *Excerpta Medical/EMBASE,* the RSNA Index of Imaging Literature, *MEDLINE/PubMed (Index Medicus),* MEDLINE/MEDLARS, SciSearch, Research Alert, and Neuroscience Citation Index.

PROGRAM OBJECTIVE:
The goal of Neuroimaging Clinics of North America is to keep practicing radiologists and radiology residents up to date with current clinical practice in radiology by providing timely articles reviewing the state of the art in patient care.

TARGET AUDIENCE
Practicing radiologists, radiology residents, and other healthcare professionals who utilize neuroimaging findings to provide patient care.

LEARNING OBJECTIVES
Upon completion of this activity, participants will be able to:
1. Discuss postoperative spine complications
2. Explain postoperative imaging of cancer patients
3. Review techniques for optimized postoperative spine imaging.

ACCREDITATION
The Elsevier Office of Continuing Medical Education (EOCME) is accredited by the Accreditation Council for Continuing Medical Education (ACCME) to provide continuing medical education for physicians.

The EOCME designates this enduring material for a maximum of 15 *AMA PRA Category 1 Credit*(s)™. Physicians should claim only the credit commensurate with the extent of their participation in the activity.

All other health care professionals requesting continuing education credit for this enduring material will be issued a certificate of participation.

DISCLOSURE OF CONFLICTS OF INTEREST
The EOCME assesses conflict of interest with its instructors, faculty, planners, and other individuals who are in a position to control the content of CME activities. All relevant conflicts of interest that are identified are thoroughly vetted by EOCME for fair balance, scientific objectivity, and patient care recommendations. EOCME is committed to providing its learners with CME activities that promote improvements or quality in healthcare and not a specific proprietary business or a commercial interest.

The planning committee, staff, authors and editors listed below have identified no financial relationships or relationships to products or devices they or their spouse/life partner have with commercial interest related to the content of this CME activity:
Roi M. Bittane, MD; Michael K. Brooks, MD, MPH; Idoia Corcuera-Solano, MD; Esther E. Coronel, MD; Simon Daniel, MD; Kimberly Dao, MD; Amichai Erdfarb, MD; Jeffrey Gnerre, MD; Kristen Helm; Brynne Hunter; Nikhil K. Jain, MD, MBA; Vivek Joshi, MD; Sudhir Kathuria, MD; Ruby J. Lien, MD; Joseph P. Mazzie, DO; Anne Marie McLellan, DO; Jill McNair; Todd Miller, MD; Suresh K. Mukherji, MD, FACR; Ryan Murtagh, MD; A. Orlando Ortiz, MD, MBA, FACR; Jeffrey S. Ross, MD; Karthikeyan Subramaniam; John Vassallo; Morgan C. Willson, BSc, MSc, MD; Richard Zampolin, MD.

The planning committee, staff, authors and editors listed below have identified financial relationships or relationships to products or devices they or their spouse/life partner have with commercial interest related to the content of this CME activity:
Alexandre B. de Moura, MD is a consultant/advisor for Stryker.
Lawrence N. Tanenbaum, MD is on speakers bureau for GE Healthcare and Siemens Corporation.

UNAPPROVED/OFF-LABEL USE DISCLOSURE
The EOCME requires CME faculty to disclose to the participants:
1. When products or procedures being discussed are off-label, unlabelled, experimental, and/or investigational (not US Food and Drug Administration (FDA) approved); and
2. Any limitations on the information presented, such as data that are preliminary or that represent ongoing research, interim analyses, and/or unsupported opinions. Faculty may discuss information about pharmaceutical agents that is outside of FDA-approved labelling. This information is intended solely for CME and is not intended to promote off-label use of these medications. If you have any questions, contact the medical affairs department of the manufacturer for the most recent prescribing information.

TO ENROLL
To enroll in the *Neuroimaging Clinics of North America* Continuing Medical Education program, call customer service at 1-800-654-2452 or sign up online at http://www.theclinics.com/home/cme. The CME program is available to subscribers for an additional annual fee of $235 USD.

METHOD OF PARTICIPATION
In order to claim credit, participants must complete the following:
1. Complete enrolment as indicated above.
2. Read the activity.
3. Complete the CME Test and Evaluation. Participants must achieve a score of 70% on the test. All CME Tests and Evaluations must be completed online.

CME INQUIRIES/SPECIAL NEEDS
For all CME inquiries or special needs, please contact elsevierCME@elsevier.com.

NEUROIMAGING CLINICS OF NORTH AMERICA

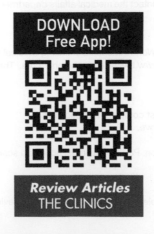

DOWNLOAD
Free App!

Review Articles
THE CLINICS

NOW AVAILABLE FOR YOUR iPhone and iPad

Contributors

CONSULTING EDITOR

SURESH K. MUKHERJI, MD, FACR
Professor and Chairman; W.F. Patenge
Endowed Chair, Department of Radiology,
Michigan State University, East Lansing,
Michigan

EDITOR

A. ORLANDO ORTIZ, MD, MBA, FACR
Chairman, Department of Radiology,
Winthrop-University Hospital, Mineola,
New York

AUTHORS

ROI M. BITTANE, MD
Department of Radiology, Winthrop-University
Hospital, Mineola, New York

MICHAEL K. BROOKS, MD, MPH
Attending Musculoskeletal Radiologist,
Division of Musculoskeletal and Interventional
Radiology; Assistant Professor of Clinical
Radiology, Stony Brook University School
of Medicine, Stony Brook, New York

ANTONIO E. CASTELLVI, MD
Foundation for Orthopaedic Research and
Education, Florida Orthopaedic Institute,
Tampa, Florida

IDOIA CORCUERA-SOLANO, MD
Department of Neuroradiology, Icahn School
of Medicine at Mount Sinai, New York,
New York

ESTHER E. CORONEL, MD
Department of Radiology, Winthrop-University
Hospital, Mineola, New York

SIMON DANIEL, MD
Department of Neuroradiology, Icahn School
of Medicine at Mount Sinai, New York,
New York

KIMBERLY DAO, MD
Division of Internal Medicine, University
of Pittsburgh Medical Center, Montefiore
Hospital, Pittsburgh, Pennsylvania

ALEXANDRE B. DE MOURA, MD
Assistant Clinical Professor of Orthopaedic
Surgery, NYU School of Medicine, New York,
New York

AMICHAI ERDFARB, MD
Assistant Professor of Clinical Radiology,
Division of Diagnostic and Interventional
Neuroradiology, Department of Radiology,
Montefiore Medical Center, Albert Einstein
College of Medicine, Bronx, New York

JEFFREY GNERRE, MD
Radiology Resident, New York Medical
College at Westchester Medical Center,
Valhalla, New York

NIKHIL K. JAIN, MD, MBA
Department of Radiology, Winthrop-University
Hospital, Mineola, New York

VIVEK JOSHI, MD
Department of Neuroradiology, Icahn School
of Medicine at Mount Sinai, New York,
New York

SUDHIR KATHURIA, MD
Assistant Professor of Radiology and
Neurosurgery, The Russell H. Morgan
Department of Radiology and Radiological
Science, Johns Hopkins Hospital, Baltimore,
Maryland

RUBY J. LIEN, MD
Attending Neuroradiologist, Department
of Radiology, Winthrop-University Hospital,
Mineola, New York

JOSEPH P. MAZZIE, DO
Program Director, Department of Radiology,
Winthrop-University Hospital, Mineola,
New York; Attending Musculoskeletal
Radiologist, Division of Musculoskeletal and
Interventional Radiology; Assistant Professor
of Clinical Radiology, Stony Brook University
School of Medicine, Stony Brook, New York

ANNE MARIE MCLELLAN, DO
Department of Neuroradiology, Icahn School
of Medicine at Mount Sinai, New York,
New York

TODD MILLER, MD
Associate Professor of Clinical Radiology,
Division of Diagnostic and Interventional
Neuroradiology, Department of Radiology,
Montefiore Medical Center, Albert Einstein
College of Medicine, Bronx, New York

RYAN MURTAGH, MD, MBA
Director of Spine Imaging; Associate Professor
of Radiology, University of South Florida,
Tampa, Florida

A. ORLANDO ORTIZ, MD, MBA, FACR
Chairman, Department of Radiology,
Winthrop-University Hospital, Mineola,
New York

JEFFREY S. ROSS, MD
Professor, Department of Neuroradiology,
Barrow Neurologic Institute, St Joseph's
Hospital and Medical Center, Phoenix, Arizona

LAWRENCE N. TANENBAUM, MD
Department of Neuroradiology, Icahn
School of Medicine at Mount Sinai, New York,
New York

MORGAN C. WILLSON, MD
Department of Radiology, Foothills Medical
Center, Calgary, Alberta, Canada

RICHARD ZAMPOLIN, MD
Assistant Professor of Clinical Radiology,
Division of Diagnostic and Interventional
Neuroradiology, Department of Radiology,
Montefiore Medical Center, Albert Einstein
College of Medicine, Bronx, New York

Contents

myeloma comprise most of these lesions. Management of spinal tumors includes surgical decompression with stabilization, (neo) adjuvant chemotherapy and radiation therapy, curettage, bone grafting, bone marrow replacement, and palliative treatment with vertebral augmentation. Pre- and postoperative imaging plays a critical role in the diagnosis and management of patients with spinal tumors. This article reviews postoperative imaging of the spine, including imaging protocols, immediate and long-term routine imaging findings, and emergent findings in symptomatic patients.

Although imaging plays a critical role and has become an integral part in preprocedure evaluation of osteoporotic patients at risk of compression fracture, many treated patients undergo follow-up imaging, for reasons ranging from potential procedure-related complications to development of new symptoms after initial improvement after successful vertebral augmentation (VA). Although imaging is frequently obtained for evaluation of these patients, there is a general lack of knowledge about imaging characteristics of treated vertebrae. This article reviews various indications for post-VA imaging, the appearance of augmented spine on imaging, and the important complications associated with the VA procedure.

Few tasks in imaging are more challenging than that of optimizing evaluations of the instrumented spine. The authors describe how applying fundamental and more advanced principles to postoperative spine computed tomography and magnetic resonance examinations mitigates the challenges associated with metal implants and significantly improves image quality and consistency. Newer and soon-to-be-available enhancements should provide improved visualization of tissues and hardware as multispectral imaging sequences continue to develop.

Imaging evaluation of postoperative spinal infection is challenging. A systematic approach and keen understanding of multimodality imaging techniques, as well as knowledge of the patient's surgical procedure and clinical presentation, are critical for the radiologist to render an accurate diagnosis. Because of the overlap between diagnostic imaging findings in the postoperative spine and the infected spine, in those situations in which the index of clinical suspicion for spine infection is high, then immediate consideration ought to be given to performing a spine biopsy.

Postoperative spine paraspinal fluid collections can present a management dilemma to both radiologists and surgeons. Although many of these collections present as incidental findings and are unrelated to the presenting signs and symptoms that led to the imaging study, certain collections in the context of the appropriate clinical scenario may require additional evaluation and even emergent intervention. This article reviews those collections that are most frequently encountered and suggests management strategies that may assist in the evaluation and management of the patient.

Foreword

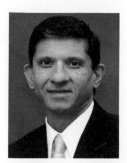

Suresh K. Mukherji, MD, FACR
Consulting Editor

This issue of *Neuroimaging Clinics* is on the very challenging and perplexing topic of postoperative spine imaging. These are clearly studies that I try to avoid; however, it is obvious that the interpreting radiologist must possess an understanding of the procedure that was performed, the normal postoperative appearance, and potential complications to provide value to patient care.

Fortunately, we have a world expert to help us understand this topic. Orlando Ortiz is one of the most accomplished neuroradiologists that specialize in this field. I have known Orlando for over twenty years and have been impressed with his expertise, accomplishments, and, mostly, his congeniality. He truly is one of the nicest and most

humble people that I have ever met and I sincerely thank him for being our editor for this very important issue. I also thank him for assembling such an outstanding group of authors. Finally, I thank the authors for their superb contributions that have inspired me to read all of the postoperative spine studies that I can find!

Suresh K. Mukherji, MD, FACR
Department of Radiology
Michigan State University
East Lansing, MI 48824, USA

E-mail address:
Mukherji@rad.msu.edu

Neuroimag Clin N Am 24 (2014) xi
http://dx.doi.org/10.1016/j.nic.2014.02.002
1052-5149/14/$ – see front matter © 2014 Published by Elsevier Inc.

Preface

Postoperative Spine Imaging and Evaluation

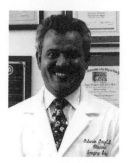

A. Orlando Ortiz, MD, MBA, FACR
Editor

The very mention of postoperative spine imaging and evaluation precipitates eye rolling among my colleagues. It is one of those areas in radiology where the study remains the longest in the imaging cue. The patient is often uncomfortable, in pain, and somewhat confused. The surgeon or operator is uncertain of what has happened. The prior studies are often missing or performed at another institution or outside imaging facility. Yet, in the midst of these obstacles and challenges, there are opportunities to assist both the patient and the referring clinician.

A working knowledge of commonly performed spine surgeries and spine interventions facilitates a thorough evaluation of the postoperative spine. The interpreting radiologist should possess a reasonable understanding of the procedure that was performed. A discussion with the referring clinician may not only clarify exactly what was done, but also allow the referring clinician to express their specific concerns about the case. An understanding of the "normal" imaging appearances of the postoperative spine is paramount. The radiology report is critical and should help both the referring clinician and the patient. Poorly worded or circumscribed reports are of limited value and may serve as fodder for medicolegal issues. With the advent of patient portals, these reports must be appropriately rendered so as not to confuse the patient. Last, in this new era of value-based imaging, appropriate diagnostic imaging and reporting take on potentially more meaningful use.

This issue of *Neuroimaging Clinics* deals with postoperative spine imaging and evaluation. I thank all of the authors for emphasizing the practical aspects in this area of spine care. The initial articles update the reader on current spine surgery techniques and approaches, including fusion and motion-sparing spine instrumentation. A spine surgeon shares his concerns over the information that he requires after ordering an imaging examination in an operated patient. This concept also applies to postprocedure imaging in patients who have undergone percutaneous vertebral augmentation or are being treated for cancer that involves the spinal axis. An awareness of potential treatment-related complications that might occur in any of these patient groups is very important. Given the diagnostic challenges of adequately imaging postoperative spine patients, emerging techniques for artifact reduction are introduced and reviewed. Specific situations in which our expertise is sought out include the management of postoperative fluid collections and spine infection. It is, therefore, my hope that readers will find this issue of particular practical value in addressing what is initially perceived as a complex case mix.

A. Orlando Ortiz, MD, MBA, FACR
Department of Radiology
Winthrop-University Hospital
259 1st Street
Mineola, NY 11501, USA

E-mail address:
oortiz@winthrop.org

Neuroimag Clin N Am 24 (2014) xiii
http://dx.doi.org/10.1016/j.nic.2014.02.001
1052-5149/14/$ – see front matter © 2014 Published by Elsevier Inc.

neuroimaging.theclinics.com

Imaging of Lumbar Spine Fusion

Richard Zampolin, MD, Amichai Erdfarb, MD,
Todd Miller, MD*

KEYWORDS

- Lumbar spine fusion • Arthrodesis • Imaging • Complications

KEY POINTS

- An awareness of the preoperative imaging, the surgical technique and history, and the set of clinical problems and imaging findings most likely to occur at specific postoperative time intervals will greatly improve the accuracy and value of imaging in reports patients with lumbar fusion.
- Fusion surgeries can be categorized into anterior, lateral, and posterior approaches, each with advantages and disadvantages.
- Outcomes studies have not demonstrated a specific benefit of one type over another.
- Surgical exploration is the gold standard for definitive fusion assessment. Thin-section computed tomography with multiplanar reconstruction is the most sensitive and specific imaging modality to detect pseudarthrosis.

INTRODUCTION

Lumbar spinal fusion, or arthrodesis, has been performed since 1911 when it was originally described by Drs Fred Albee and Russell Hibbs, who were the first to use autologous bone graft for spinal stabilization.[1,2] As shown in **Figs. 1** and **2**, decorticated, bleeding cortical surfaces are surgically created and osseous substrates are implanted in the disc space (interbody) or adjacent to the facet joints in a space termed the posterolateral gutter as the necessary components for successful fusion or bone healing. The process creates a physiologic environment favorable for bone formation, which is intended to limit motion of the treated spinal segment.[3]

Fusion surgeries are performed to prevent motion of a single or multiple spinal segments, to alleviate pain or prevent neurologic compromise (**Box 1**). Reviews and prospective randomized trials have demonstrated improved patient outcomes when successful fusion operations have been performed.[4–7] Immediate stabilization improves the chance of successful arthrodesis.[8] Before instrumentation was popularized, this was achieved with bracing or bed rest.[9] Multilevel fusions were soon recognized as producing lower success rates for solid fusion and increased rates of pseudarthrosis. Instrumented fusion was designed to address this lower success rate with multilevel procedures. Over time, instrumented fusion was shown to provide effective immediate immobilization of the fused segment, theoretically increasing the likelihood of successful fusion for single-level procedures as had been shown for multilevel procedures. Implants, however, do not take the place of physiologic bony fusion, and are not designed to provide segmental immobility beyond the period during which true osseous fusion forms.[10] Current practice favors the combination of decorticated, bleeding osseous surfaces

Division of Diagnostic and Interventional Neuroradiology, Department of Radiology, Montefiore Medical Center, Albert Einstein College of Medicine, 111 East 210th Street, Bronx, NY 10467, USA
* Corresponding author.
E-mail address: tmiller@montefiore.org

Neuroimag Clin N Am 24 (2014) 269–286
http://dx.doi.org/10.1016/j.nic.2014.01.004
1052-5149/14/$ – see front matter © 2014 Elsevier Inc. All rights reserved.

neuroimaging.theclinics.com

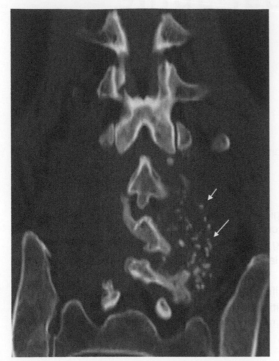

Fig. 1. Bone substrate. Immediate postoperative coronal CT scan with morselized bone fragments (*arrows*).

and implanted substrate with spinal instrumentation, to provide early internal stabilization and thus allow for eventual complete osseous fusion, as shown in **Fig. 3**.

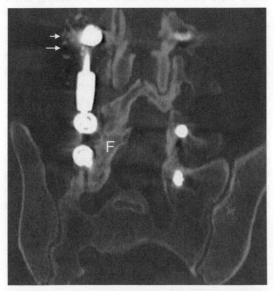

Fig. 2. Comparison of fusion with substrate. Recent postoperative CT coronal scan shows bone-graft material from a revision surgery (*arrows*). Compare with solidly fused graft from prior surgery (F).

> **Box 1**
> **Instability**
>
> Segmental instability: Loss of motion stiffness such that force application to the motion segment produces greater displacement than would be seen in normal structures, resulting in a painful condition that has the potential for progressive deformity and neurologic damage.[11]

INDICATIONS

Spine-related pain complaints are common and have several potential causes (**Box 2**). The decision to operate on the spine to relieve pain is deferred until more conservative treatment methods fail to provide a therapeutic benefit. The broadest indications for elective spinal arthrodesis are pain or instability that threatens neurologic function.

Scoliosis correction is a broad category that is not necessarily a fusion, and is beyond the scope of this article. Instability at the level of the disc and facet joints results in a cascade of degeneration leading to chronic low back pain and anatomic derangement. Disc removal and segmental arthrodesis have been used to address this problem. There are also acute clinical scenarios, such as those caused by acute spinal cord compression resulting in myelopathy, nerve root compression resulting in severe extremity pain and weakness, or cauda equina syndrome, which often necessitate immediate surgical intervention.

PRIMARY VERSUS SECONDARY FUSION

Primary fusion surgeries are performed on the group of patients thought to be suffering from low back pain who have segmental instability, but do not have demonstrable focal neural compression or spinal deformity. In this group of patients the rates of interbody fusion have dramatically increased, although the evidence to support which approach is best remains unclear.[12–15] The general surgical approaches for fusion are described in **Box 3**.

Secondary instrumented fusions result from surgeries designed primarily to accomplish decompression of the thecal sac or nerve roots. When posterolateral fusion is not possible, or instability is likely, instrumented fusion is added to the decompression. When the decompression limits available posterior elements that serve as posterolateral fusion surface area, instrumented posterior fusion or interbody fusions are

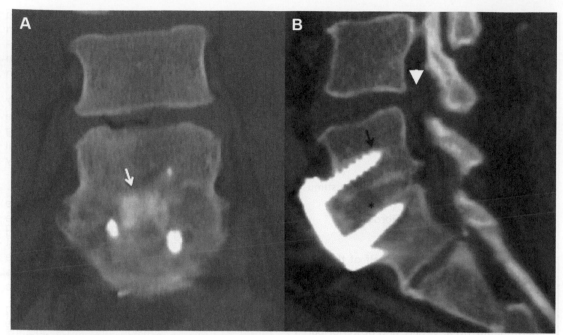

Fig. 3. Solid anterior lumbar interbody fusion. (*A*) Coronal reformatted image from computed tomography (CT) scan shows interbody graft incorporated into endplate (*arrow*). (*B*) Sagittal reformatted image from CT scan shows anterior plate and screws (*black arrow*) with graft well incorporated into endplates (*black asterisk*). Unfused level above has developed disc protrusion (*white arrowhead*).

performed. Iatrogenic instability from bilateral facetectomies as part of a decompression may cause instability that would lead to kyphotic deformity or accelerated degeneration. Secondary fusions are additionally performed as part of these decompression surgeries.

USE OF HARDWARE

The rate of instrumented fusion increased rapidly as evidence for increased arthrodesis rates with instrumentation and the development of improved

spinal hardware occurred simultaneously.[15,20] Instrumentation in the current practice of lumbar fusion consists of pedicle screws, plates, rods, and intervertebral implants (hollow cages or solid ramps), which all act as internal fixation devices to immediately limit segmental motion from the time of surgery and are thought to improve the rates of subsequent osseous fusion. In addition, interbody grafts and devices increase disc-space height and can act to immediately increase foraminal and canal area by separating pedicles and putting traction on hypertrophied ligaments, as is shown in **Fig. 4**.[21–24]

SURGICAL METHODS

An understanding of the specific surgical approach allows an appreciation of the expected postoperative imaging appearance of the surgical bed as well as the possible complications, as shown in **Figs. 5** and **6** (**Box 4**). The surgical approach to spinal fusion can be thought of as anterior, posterior, or lateral. Each approach is used to achieve arthrodesis while avoiding injury to the thecal sac and exiting nerves. Traditional open surgical methods still predominate, although newer minimally invasive methods are growing in popularity for specific indications. Outcomes studies have not demonstrated a specific benefit

---

Box 2
Etiology of spine pain

Common

Muscle strain

Disc degeneration

Facet arthropathy

Spinal stenosis

Less Common

Trauma

Infection

Neoplasm

Instability (degenerative, traumatic, iatrogenic)

Box 3
General anatomic approaches to spinal fusion and their relative advantages

Anterior:

- Broad access to the anterior disc space allowing for complete anterior and central disc removal
- Optimization of fusion cage size and surface contact with the osseous endplates
- Restoration of full disc height
- Improved internal stabilization, which stimulates osseous fusion
- Decreased risk of epidural fibrosis[16]

Lateral:

- Wide access to the anterior half of the disc space allowing for a thorough discectomy, and placement of a large implant under adequate traction[17]
- Avoids violation and direct retraction of the peritoneum, great vessels, and posterior paraspinal muscles
- Shorter operative time in comparison with laparoscopic anterior lumbar interbody fusion

Posterior:

- Direct access to the spinal canal and neural elements allowing for complete decompression of the thecal sac and nerve roots, as well as some disc height restoration and a fairly complete discectomy[18]
- Open access to the posterior elements facilitates optimal placement of spinal instrumentation such as pedicle screws and bridging rods
- Posterior dissection avoids risks of abdominal visceral injury

---

of one type over another.[13] Anterior and lateral access is preferred when disc degeneration, endplate changes, and loss of disc height predominate without the need for posterior or lateral decompression and fusion. In cases of focal posterior or lateral disc herniations and/or significant spinal stenosis, a posterior approach and decompression is necessary. Based on decreased operative time and blood loss, a convincing argument is made for stand-alone interbody fusion in those patients who do not require posterior decompression.[19]

INTRAOPERATIVE IMAGING

There is currently no standard practice for image guidance in the operating room. Imaging for instrumented lumbar fusion is performed on a spectrum from no image guidance (based on anatomic landmarks, neurophysiology, and tactile response) to full 3-dimensional real-time computer-assisted image guidance using an O-arm computed tomography (CT) and pedicle-screw tracking systems as shown in **Figs. 7** and **8**. Use of intraoperative fluoroscopy is the mainstay of clinical practice, along with a growing use of an O-arm CT guidance system. Several studies have demonstrated improved accuracy of pedicle-screw placement using image guidance to verify placement of screw trajectories.[27–29] Newer systems using preoperative CT, computer registration, and modeling provide real-time tracking of implant placement during the operations.[27,29]

POSTOPERATIVE IMAGING

Lumbar CT may be performed at the conclusion of a lumbar fusion surgery to evaluate hardware placement, spinal alignment, or a complication. Despite the use of intraoperative image guidance, these studies are sometimes required to precisely document placement of spinal instrumentation, verify postprocedure spinal alignment, and exclude complications. Following the immediate postoperative imaging any additional imaging is generally unnecessary, as imaging of the healing spine can be misleading.[30–35] Normal postoperative imaging findings such as small epidural collections (with and without hemorrhage), granulation tissue, osteoclastic bone resorption (especially in the setting of using recombinant human bone morphogenic protein [rhBMP][24,36]) all can be misinterpreted as abnormal during the period of normal healing, especially on magnetic resonance (MR) imaging.[31,33–35] However, if a clinical problem arises, such as worsening pain beyond the expected postoperative pain, new neurologic deficit, or clinical signs of infection, imaging may be required (**Boxes 5** and **6**).

Postoperative MR Imaging

There is no evidence-based guideline for evaluation of postoperative symptoms. In the absence of trauma, when faced with a new neurologic deficit, worsening pain, or possible infection, the superior tissue contrast provided by MR imaging allows identification of hematomas, pseudomeningoceles, and infection.[30–35,37–49] Modern implants have fewer ferromagnetic artifacts that plagued the images of older devices. Most immediate postoperative collections are seromas, which may

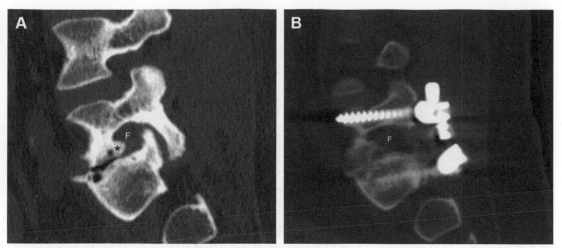

Fig. 4. Foraminal enlargement. (*A*) Sagittal view from CT scan shows the neural foramen (F) narrowed by lost disc space height (compare with level above) and annular osteophyte (*asterisk*). (*B*) Sagittal postoperative view shows enlarged foramen (F).

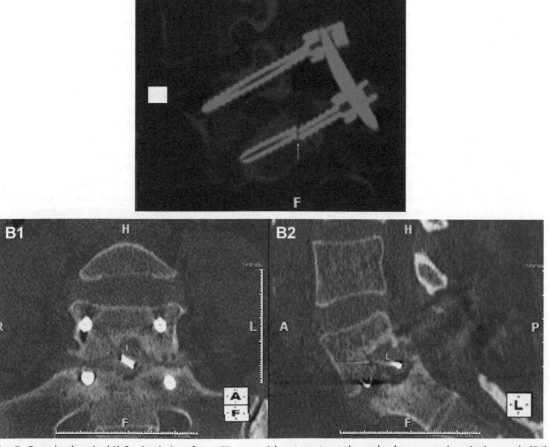

Fig. 5. Pseudarthrosis. (*A*) Sagittal view from CT scan without contrast shows broken screw (*vertical arrow*). (*B1*) Coronal reformat from CT scan shows lucency around cage (L). (*B2*) Sagittal reformat from CT shows lucency around cage (L).

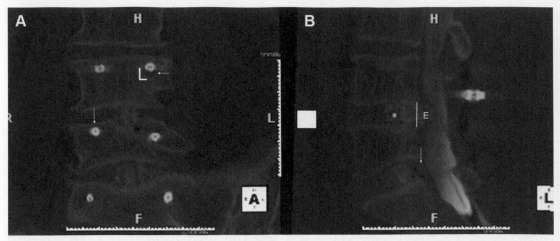

Fig. 6. Ejected cage. (A) Coronal view from CT myelogram shows 2-level fusion with cages. Screw loosening is shown by horizontal arrow (L). Vertical arrow indicates the well-incorporated screw. (B) Sagittal view shows ejected cage (E) more than 2 mm past posterior margin of disc annulus (*vertical line*). Level below shows normally located graft, which does not extend past posterior annulus marked by vertical arrow. Lucent lines around cages indicate failure to incorporate.

have a complex appearance difficult to distinguish from early infection.[42,44] Dynamic CT myelography may be helpful in differentiating a communicating cerebrospinal fluid (CSF) collection from a seroma.[43]

Postoperative CT

Surgical exploration has been the gold standard for the assessment of arthrodesis.[50,51] The process of choosing the preferred noninvasive imaging marker has evolved over time.[19,52] Owing to the intrinsic cost and availability benefits, flexion and extension plain films were often used to evaluate for evidence of fusion and signs of motion at the fusion level, findings consistent with incomplete fusion, or fusion failure and pseudarthrosis, depending on the timing of imaging.[22] The value of MR imaging in this context is inherently limited by susceptibility artifact, which degrades fine bony detail, often obscuring the imaging findings of osseous fusion. CT scanning provides superior 3-dimensional fine bony detail and multiplanar reconstructions for evaluation of progressive arthrodesis, as shown in **Figs. 9 and 10**.[53,54]

FUSION ASSESSMENT

Fusion occurs in a series of stages, which can be readily identified on thin-section CT scans.[22] Trabecular bridging is a marker for fusion and

has been detailed previously.[55] Lucency or cystic changes adjacent to hardware should be absent.[56] Such lucency surrounding the hardware signifies persistent motion at the bone-hardware interface, reaction to rhBMP, or infection. These findings may be subtle and can be misinterpreted as metal-associated photon loss (appearing as a lucent line) surrounding the hardware. Specific high-spatial-frequency CT algorithms and multiplanar thin-section reconstructions can improve detection of this finding.[21,35,57–62] Trabecular bridging often first occurs outside of the interbody implant. Centrally interrupted bony trabeculation within the interbody space or misalignment of these trabeculations suggests motion, delayed union, and possible early pseudarthrosis formation, as shown in **Fig. 11**.[22,63–66] A lack of mature trabeculations crossing the disc space at 24 months represents failed fusion and, likely, pseudarthrosis formation.[67] Alternative maneuvers such as extension CT scanning have been devised to help improve the sensitivity and specificity.[68]

The imaging evaluation of posterolateral fusion is different from interbody fusion. The posterolateral fusion mass starts out as a conglomerate of morselized bone fragments, which are packed along the lateral gutters between the transverse processes and adjacent to the facet joints. Over time the discrete bone fragments of this mass begin to fuse into a solid bone bridge between the facets and transverse processes. If this

---

Box 4
Lumbar spine fusion techniques

Posterolateral Lumbar Fusion (PLF)

Technique (Hibbs[2])

- Midline incision, retraction of the paraspinal muscles
- Decortication and placement of osseous substrate
- Instrumentation with pedicle-screw placement may be performed
- Laminectomy with posterior decompression may be performed depending on the specific pathologic circumstance[35–37]

Complications

- Fibrosis adjacent the exiting nerve roots or thecal sac
- Hardware or bone-graft material impingement of the neural elements
- Dural tears

Posterolateral Lumbar Interbody Fusion (PLIF) (See Fig. 2)

Technique (Cloward[37,38])

- Thecal sac and nerve roots freed and retracted to the midline
- Annulotomy and complete discectomy
- Removal of central disc material and cartilaginous endplates
- Implant to restore disc space height and optimize stimulus for osseous fusion

Complications

- Retraction damage to the conus or exiting nerves
- Dural tears
- Fibrosis that can result in chronic pain[8,39]
- Postoperative radiculopathy rates of up to 13%[37,40,41]
- Postoperative instability and posterior migration of the fusion construct[3,25,29]

Transforaminal Lumbar Interbody Fusion (TLIF)

Technique (Harms and Rolinger[5,42,43])

- Placement of pedicle screws above and below the abnormal disc segment
- Distraction to provide space for implant[8,44]
- Unilateral facetectomy and mobilization of the exiting nerve
- Preservation of the contralateral laminae and spinous processes
- Complete discectomy, bone-graft placement, and cage implantation

Complications

- Cage migration rates of 1.17%[11,42] (See Fig.3)
- Fibrosis from retraction and passage of fusion implant through transforaminal space

Anterior Lumbar Interbody Fusion (ALIF)

Technique (Burns[45])

- Parasagittal lower abdominal incision, retraction of the peritoneal contents, lumbosacral prevertebral neural elements, and great vessels to access the midline anterior lumbar spine
- Microsurgical modification of the ALIF developed by Mayer enters through the rectus muscles to the preperitoneal space[13,46]
- Middle section of the annulus resected with the nucleus pulposus
- Cartilaginous endplates resected to level of bleeding osseous endplates
- Cage implant is fitted into the anterior disc space to restore disc height

Complications

- Vascular injury, perforated viscera, and damage to the lumbar plexus[15,47,48]
- Incontinence, sexual dysfunction, and retrograde ejaculation[17,26]
- Abdominal wall hernias
- Deep venous thrombosis

Extreme Lateral Lumbar Interbody Fusion (XLIF)

Technique (Ozgur[19,49])

- Lateral flank incisions used to access the retroperitoneal space
- Blunt dissection used to reach to the psoas muscle, which is split in anterior third
- Discectomy is performed similar to the ALIF technique, with preservation of the posterior annulus and creation of a wide space for an anterior fusion implant

Complications

- Vascular damage
- Psoas hematoma
- Lumbar plexus nerve damage
- Abdominal wall hernias
- Deep venous thrombosis[24,33]

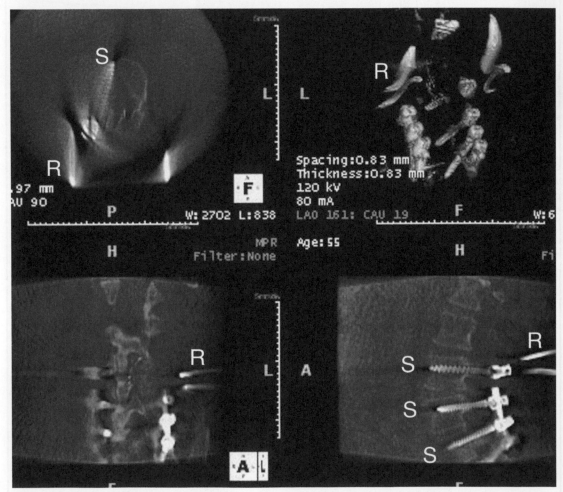

Fig. 7. Intraoperative O-arm CT. Four-panel composite shows limited contrast images with metallic beam-hardening artifacts caused by low-dose scan. Hardware (pedicle screw, S) placements are well demonstrated to allow immediate revision if necessary. Retractors are in place as wound remains open (R).

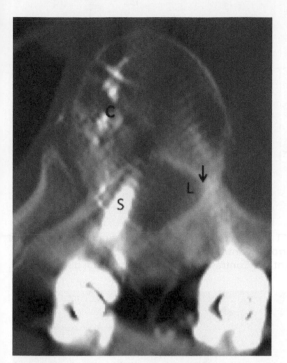

Fig. 8. Misplaced pedicle screw. Intraoperative CT scan shows pedicle screw (S) violating medial boarder of pedicle (*arrow*) within the lateral recess (L). This patient was osteoporotic, and the screw tracts were prepared with cement (C) to improve screw purchase.

coalition of the bony morsels fails to occur within 24 months postoperatively or a discrete discontinuity is apparent in the bony bridge, failed or incomplete fusion has occurred, as shown in **Fig. 12.**[69,70]

Box 5
Postoperative spine imaging indications

Within days of surgery (acute phase): Surveillance, or unexpectedly intense pain or a new neurologic deficit

Within first 2 months of surgery (early subacute phase): Surveillance, or because of insufficient postoperative recovery and persistent pain

Within first year (late subacute phase): Surveillance, or because of persistent complaints of patient discomfort

After several pain-free years (chronic): Return of pain either in a similar distribution to preoperative pain, or in a different distribution

Surveillance is used to ascertain hardware position or progression of osseous fusion.

Box 6
Postoperative evaluation

Confirmation of level treated in comparison with preoperative imaging

Alterations of spinal anatomy: alignment, disc space height, decompression of canal and foramina

Unexpected findings: hematoma, fluid collection, foreign bodies

Assessment of surgical hardware:

Interbody implant: 2 mm from posterior margin of vertebral body[21,37]

Pedicle screw:

Centered in the pedicle

No cortical breach or vascular contact

Aligned with the superior endplate of the vertebral body or offset to facilitate placement[37,38]

Subsidence is the migration of the fusion cage through the osseous endplate (>3 mm) and the associated loss of the surgically established interbody height.[35,71,72] This phenomenon is important to recognize, as it can lead to failed surgical outcomes and is thought to occur at rates of approximately 14% with rhBMP-2 usage.[71] In the past, subsidence was more difficult to detect with stainless-steel interbody cages, which produce extensive artifact on both CT and MR imaging, and were more likely to result in subsidence because of their rigidity.[21] These rigid stainless-steel cages have been replaced with bioactive titanium and synthetic implants such as the polyetheretherketone (PEEK) cages, which have biomechanical properties more similar to that of cortical bone, are bioactive, and generate little imaging artifact.[73]

Various types of bone-graft material (autografts and allografts) and stimulating factors such as rhBMP are used to simulate osseous growth between the vertebral bodies. Although controversy exists in the literature about when to use rhBMP given its high cost, several investigators have demonstrated that the use of rhBMP provided outcomes similar to those for iliac autografts, and avoided morbidity associated with graft harvest.[70] A randomized controlled trial demonstrated improved safety, clinical efficacy, and cost-effectiveness of rhBMP-2 compared with iliac crest bone grafting in patients older than 60 years requiring lumbar fusion.[74]

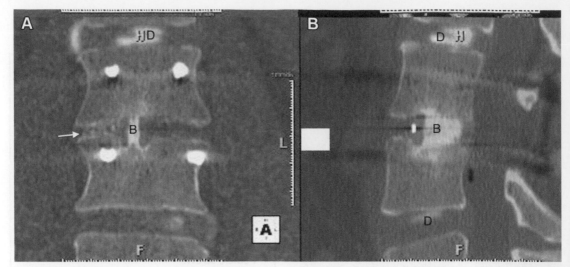

Fig. 9. Solid interbody fusion. (*A*) Coronal view from CT after discogram shows solidly bridging bone across implant (B), and additional bone bridging disk space (*arrow*). Contrast is seen in the discs from discogram (D). (*B*) Sagittal view shows solid bridging bone across implant (B). Contrast is seen in the discs from discogram (D).

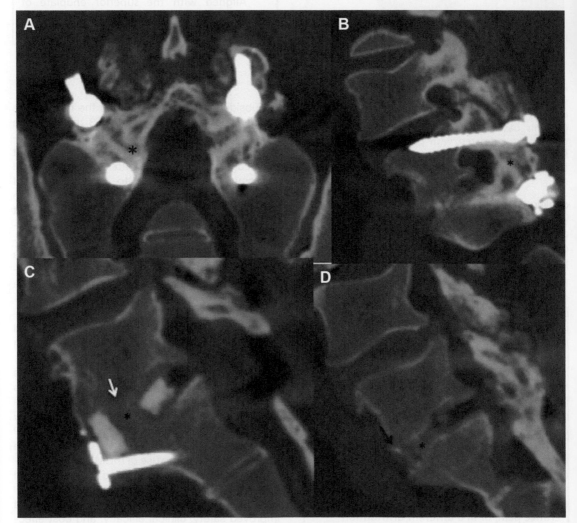

Fig. 10. Solid 360 fusion. (*A*) Coronal view from CT shows solid posterolateral fusion (*asterisk*). (*B*) Sagittal view from CT shows solid posterolateral fusion mass (*asterisk*). (*C*) Sagittal midline view form CT shows solid bridging 1082 (*arrow*) bone across implant (*asterisk*). (*D*) Parasagittal view from CT shows trabeculae bridging across disc space (*arrow*) remote from the graft (*asterisk*).

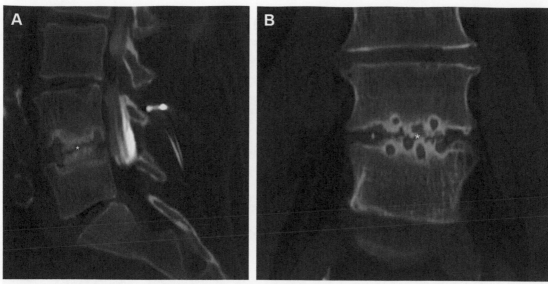

Fig. 11. Interbody pseudarthrosis. (*A*) Sagittal view from CT myelogram shows lucency across cage in horizontal plane (*asterisk*). (*B*) Coronal reformatted image from CT myelogram shows 2 cages with horizontal lucency running across (*asterisk*).

Persistent or new pain symptoms following the 12-month perioperative-healing phase will often trigger additional imaging. A significant subset (estimated to be on the order of 30% at 1 year) of patients who undergo lumbar spine surgery will suffer from persistent or recurrent low back pain or radicular symptoms despite surgical intervention.[75,76] Several umbrella terms, including failed back surgery syndrome, failed back syndrome, and postlaminectomy syndrome, are currently used to describe this condition (**Box 7**). Imaging will often reveal abnormalities not referable to the clinical syndrome, and thus must be carefully correlated with the specific clinical scenario.[77] It is important to rigorously review the existing preoperative and postoperative images while being mindful that many abnormalities will not be the cause of a patient's pain. Imaging in this context should be designed to maximize the likelihood of identifying the cause of pain while minimizing patient risk, radiation exposure, and cost.

Traditionally the first-line imaging study has been flexion and extension plain film radiography of the affected spine. These images are insensitive to subtle fusion, hardware loosening, and motion, which limits their ability to distinguish between incomplete fusion and true pseudarthrosis.[19] In addition, plain radiography does not effectively evaluate the soft tissues for entities such as epidural scar formation, recurrent disc disease, epidural abscess, or signs of chronic infection.[42]

MR Imaging

Contrast-enhanced MR imaging of the affected spinal levels can help distinguish between epidural scar formation, which enhances homogeneously, and recurrent or residual disc disease, which enhances peripherally. MR imaging also provides a detailed evaluation of the thecal sac and paraspinal soft tissues, allowing for the diagnosis of soft-tissue collections, enhancement, and arachnoiditis. Arachnoiditis may occur after surgical manipulation of the thecal sac, and has a characteristic appearance on MR imaging. Arachnoiditis typically appears as a conglomerate of adherent nerve roots centrally within the thecal sac, an empty appearance of the thecal sac secondary to nerve roots, which are displaced along the walls and adherent to the sac, and a clumped soft-tissue mass replacing the subarachnoid space secondary to fibrotic adhesions.[34]

MR imaging in this setting has several limitations, including limited bony detail and decreased sensitivity to hardware loosening and bony fusion.[78] As with CT, MR imaging is limited by hardware artifact. This limitation can be mitigated by imaging in a magnet of relatively lower field strength and by choosing appropriate acquisition parameters designed to limit artifacts based on

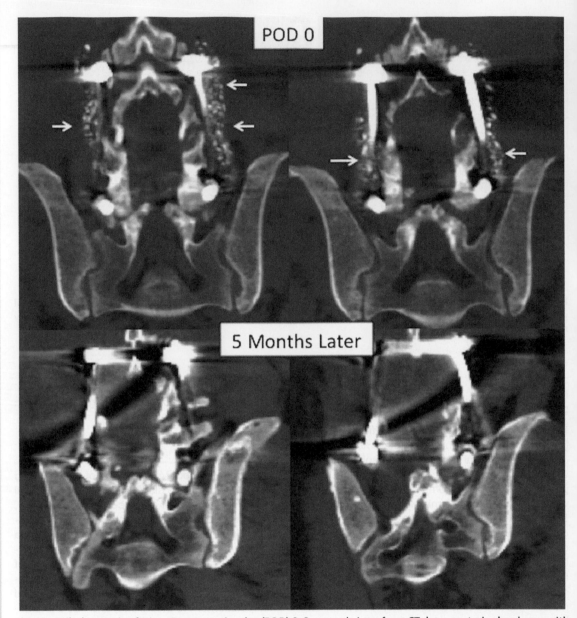

Fig. 12. Failed posterior fusion. Postoperative day (POD) 0: 2 coronal views from CT show posterior hardware with morselized bone fragments lining the lateral gutters (*arrows*). Five months later: morselized bone has been resorbed and a solid fusion has not occurred.

Box 7
Causes of failed back surgery syndrome

- Recurrent disc disease
- Incorrect level or surgery
- Epidural fibrosis
- Dural injury
- Neural injury
- Pseudarthrosis

magnetic-field inhomogeneity.[79] Not all patients can tolerate MR imaging for reasons of pain, claustrophobia, or the presence of non-MR compatible implants (older ferromagnetic cerebral aneurysm clips, incompatible pacemakers, newly placed stents, etc).

CT

CT can be an effective modality for demonstrating the course of postoperative osseous fusion (**Box 8**). Following the expected course of

---

Box 8
Signs of interbody fusion and loosening

Signs of fusion

- 3 months: increased density around and within the intervertebral implant
- 6 months: uninterrupted trabecular bony bridging from endplate to endplate
- 12+ months: dense mature trabeculations and solid cortical bone bridging the intervertebral space

Signs of hardware loosening (**Fig. 13**)

- Changes in screw orientation
- Osseous lucency/sclerosis surrounding screws
- Hardware fracture
- Pseudarthrosis
- Subsidence

---

arthrodesis, CT is a sensitive modality for identifying patients with fusion failure and pseudarthrosis.[80,81] When compared with plain radiography or MR imaging, CT can better demonstrate subtle periprosthetic lucency, a marker of hardware loosening that can be due to mechanical instability or infection. CT is also better suited to the identification of new bone formation, both between vertebral bodies and surrounding the posterior elements, allowing for an accurate assessment of fusion progression or detection of pseudarthrosis development. In addition, CT is sensitive for the formation of heterotopic bone formation secondary to the surgical intervention or abnormal postoperative stresses resulting in abnormal bone growth, which may compress neural elements and elicit pain. The limitations of CT are limited soft-tissue contrast in comparison with MR imaging, streak artifact from implanted hardware obscuring adjacent tissues, and the associated radiation exposure.

CT Myelography

CT myelography combines the benefits of conventional CT imaging (display of fine bony detail allowing for the evaluation of osseous fusion, pseudarthrosis formation, and periprosthetic lucency), while providing additional information about the thecal sac, conus contour, nerve root anatomy, and nerve roots.[82] For this examination, CT images are obtained after the intrathecal administration of contrast material, resulting in opacification of the subarachnoid space. This contrast allows direct and indirect evaluation of the intrathecal contents and extradural soft tissues. Although evaluation for the presence of arachnoiditis is currently most commonly performed with MR imaging, the various stages of nerve root inflammation and fibrosis were initially described with CT myelography.[83] Likewise, subtle thecal sac contour deformities indicating the presence of a residual or recurrent disc or epidural fibrosis can be demonstrated. CT myelography can also aid in the detection of a CSF fistula or pseudomeningocele formation.[84,85] Because of its invasive nature, there are risks associated with myelography that are not associated with noninvasive imaging, including the development of a CSF leak, headache, infection, or reaction to iodine contrast agent. Given these risks and the discomfort patients may experience during the procedure, myelography is usually reserved for those patients with contraindications to MR imaging, or cases whereby MR imaging does not answer the clinical question.

LONG-TERM SURVEILLANCE

Recurrent low back pain or radiculopathy years after spinal fusion may result from recurrent or new disease. It has been demonstrated in several studies that spinal fixation alters normal spinal biomechanics, transmitting the mechanical stresses of motion to the adjacent levels (**Box 9**).[86] This process is thought to accelerate disc and facet degeneration at adjacent spinal levels, which results in new disc herniations, listhesis, and facet hypertrophy. Ultimately this can lead to the development of spinal canal and neuroforaminal stenosis at initially unaffected levels.[87] Hardware migration or subsidence can also occur as the result of bone remodeling or long-standing hardware-related pressure erosions.[88] For example, this can result in screws, which were well encased in bone on early postoperative studies, protruding through the cortex and impinging on adjacent structures. In cases of such protruding hardware, pressure-related bursa may form, as well as damage to adjacent vessels or nerves. In instances of suboptimal osseous fusion, a chronic pseudarthrosis can result. Given this spectrum of possible long-term causes of new or recurrent lumbar spine symptoms, MR imaging is considered the best-choice imaging modality. If the clinical question remains unanswered or the MR imaging results are unclear, a subsequent scan with unenhanced CT or CT myelography may be necessary to determine a cause of the patient's symptoms and to determine a plan for therapeutic intervention.

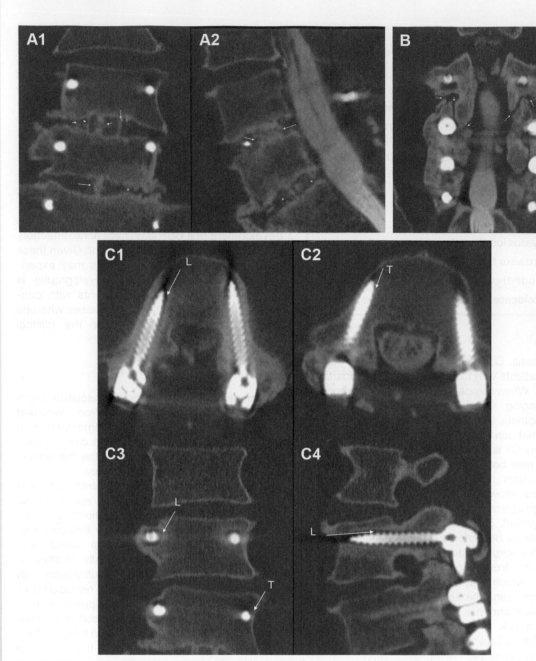

Fig. 13. Pseudarthrosis. (*A1*) Coronal views from CT scan show 3-level instrumented fusion. The arrows indicate hazy trabeculae within the cages. Asterisk shows failed crossing by bony trabeculae. (*A2*) Sagittal view from CT myelogram shows hazy crossing trabeculae (*arrows*) and failed crossing by bony ingrowth (*asterisks*). (*B*) Coronal reformatted view from CT myelogram shows interruption in the posterior fusion mass that runs across in a meandering lucent line (*arrows*) completely across the fusion mass. (*C1*) Axial view from CT myelogram shows screw with lucency and sclerotic rim caused by loosening (*arrow L*). (*C2*) Axial view from CT myelogram shows well-seated tight screw (*arrow T*). (*C3*) Coronal view from CT myelogram shows loose screw with lucent halo and sclerotic rim (*arrow L*). Compare with incorporated screw (*arrow T*). (*C4*) Sagittal reformat from CT myelogram shows loose screw with lucency and sclerotic margin (*arrow L*).

SUMMARY

Optimal imaging of lumbar spine fusion requires consideration of the timing of surgery, the type of surgical procedure, and the presenting clinical details. It is vital to have an awareness of the preoperative imaging, the surgical technique and history, and the set of clinical problems and imaging findings most likely to occur at specific postoperative time intervals. With this knowledge the care team can tailor the treatment plan to a given clinical scenario, and provide the patient with the best chances of improved clinical outcome.

REFERENCES

1. Albee FH. Transplantation of a portion of the tibia into the spine for Pott's disease: a preliminary report 1911. Clin Orthop Relat Res 2007;14–6. http://dx.doi.org/10.1097/BLO.0b013e3180686a0f.
2. Hibbs RA. A further consideration of an operation for Pott's disease of the spine: with report of cases from the service of The New York Orthopaedic Hospital. Ann Surg 1912;55(5):682–8.
3. Lipson SJ. Spinal-fusion surgery—advances and concerns. N Engl J Med 2004;350(7):643–4. http://dx.doi.org/10.1056/NEJMp038162.
4. Pearson AM, Lurie JD, Tosteson TD, et al. Who should have surgery for degenerative spondylolisthesis?: treatment effect predictors in SPORT. Spine (Phila Pa 1976) 2013. http://dx.doi.org/10.1097/BRS.0b013e3182a314d0.
5. Fritzell P, Hägg O, Wessberg P, et al, Swedish Lumbar Spine Study Group. 2001 Volvo Award Winner in Clinical Studies: Lumbar fusion versus nonsurgical treatment for chronic low back pain: a multicenter randomized controlled trial from the Swedish Lumbar Spine Study Group. Spine 2001;26(23): 2521–32. http://dx.doi.org/10.1103/PhysRevD.15. 2752 [discussion: 2532–4].
6. Djurasovic M, Glassman SD, Dimar JR, et al. Does fusion status correlate with patient outcomes in lumbar spinal fusion? Spine 2011;36(5):404–9. http://dx.doi.org/10.1097/BRS.0b013e3181fde2c4.
7. Tsutsumimoto T, Shimogata M, Yoshimura Y, et al. Union versus nonunion after posterolateral lumbar fusion: a comparison of long-term surgical outcomes in patients with degenerative lumbar spondylolisthesis. Eur Spine J 2008;17(8):1107–12. http://dx.doi.org/10.1007/s00586-008-0695-9.
8. Kornblum MB, Fischgrund JS, Herkowitz HN, et al. Degenerative lumbar spondylolisthesis with spinal stenosis: a prospective long-term study comparing fusion and pseudarthrosis. Spine 2004;29(7): 726–33 [discussion: 733–4].
9. Yee AJ, Yoo JU, Marsolais EB, et al. Use of a postoperative lumbar corset after lumbar spinal arthrodesis for degenerative conditions of the spine. A prospective randomized trial. J Bone Joint Surg Am 2008;90(10):2062–8. http://dx.doi.org/10. 2106/JBJS.G.01093.
10. Slone RM, McEnery KW, Bridwell KH, et al. Fixation techniques and instrumentation used in the thoracic, lumbar, and lumbosacral spine. Radiol Clin North Am 1995;33(2):233–65.
11. Frymoyer JW, Selby DK. Segmental instability. Rationale for treatment. Spine 1985;10(3):280–6.
12. Resnick DK, Choudhri TF, Dailey AT, et al. Guidelines for the performance of fusion procedures for degenerative disease of the lumbar spine. Part 11: interbody techniques for lumbar fusion. J Neurosurg Spine 2005;2:692–9.
13. Abdu WA, Lurie JD, Spratt KF, et al. Degenerative spondylolisthesis: does fusion method influence outcome? Four-year results of the spine patient outcomes research trial. Spine 2009;34(21):2351–60. http://dx.doi.org/10.1097/BRS.0b013e3181b8a829.
14. Tsahtsarlis A, Wood M. Minimally invasive transforaminal lumbar interbody fusion and spondylolisthesis. J Clin Neurosci 2012;19(6):858–61. http://dx. doi.org/10.1016/j.jocn.2011.10.007.
15. Babu MA, Coumans JV, Carter BS, et al. A review of lumbar spinal instrumentation: evidence and controversy. J Neurol Neurosurg Psychiatry 2011; 82(9):948–51. http://dx.doi.org/10.1136/jnnp.2010. 231860.
16. Zdeblick TA, David SM. A prospective comparison of surgical approach for anterior L4-L5 fusion: laparoscopic versus mini anterior lumbar interbody fusion. Spine 2000;25(20):2682–7.
17. Ozgur BM, Aryan HE, Pimenta L, et al. Extreme lateral interbody fusion (XLIF): a novel surgical technique for anterior lumbar interbody fusion. Spine J 2006;6(4):435–43. http://dx.doi.org/10. 1016/j.spinee.2005.08.012.
18. Branch CL. The case for posterior lumbar interbody fusion. Clin Neurosurg 1996;43:252–67.
19. McAfee PC, Boden SD, Brantigan JW, et al. Symposium: a critical discrepancy-a criteria of successful

arthrodesis following interbody spinal fusions. Spine 2001;26(3):320–34.

20. Deyo RA, Nachemson A, Mirza SK. Spinal-fusion surgery—the case for restraint. N Engl J Med 2004;350(7):722–6. http://dx.doi.org/10.1056/NEJMsb031771.

21. Rutherford EE, Tarplett LJ, Davies EM, et al. Lumbar spine fusion and stabilization: hardware, techniques, and imaging appearances. Radiographics 2007;27(6):1737–49. http://dx.doi.org/10.1148/rg.276065205.

22. Williams AL, Gornet MF, Burkus JK. CT evaluation of lumbar interbody fusion: current concepts. AJNR Am J Neuroradiol 2005;26(8):2057–66.

23. Davis W, Allouni AK, Mankad K, et al. Modern spinal instrumentation. Part 1: Normal spinal implants. Clin Radiol 2013;68(1):64–74. http://dx.doi.org/10.1016/j.crad.2012.05.001.

24. Murtagh RD, Quencer RM, Castellvi AE, et al. New techniques in lumbar spinal instrumentation: what the radiologist needs to know. Radiology 2011;260(2):317–30. http://dx.doi.org/10.1148/radiol.11101104.

25. Zhao FD, Yang W, Shan Z, et al. Cage migration after transforaminal lumbar interbody fusion and factors related to it. Orthop Surg 2012;4(4):227–32. http://dx.doi.org/10.1111/os.12004.

26. Mayer HM. A new microsurgical technique for minimally invasive anterior lumbar interbody fusion. Spine 1997;22(6):691–9 [discussion: 700].

27. Kosmopoulos V, Schizas C. Pedicle screw placement accuracy: a meta-analysis. Spine 2007;32(3):E111–20.

28. Austin MS, Vaccaro AR, Brislin B, et al. Image-guided spine surgery: a cadaver study comparing conventional open laminoforaminotomy and two image-guided techniques for pedicle screw placement in posterolateral fusion and nonfusion models. Spine 2002;27(22):2503–8. http://dx.doi.org/10.1097/01.BRS.0000031274.34509.1E.

29. Laine T, Lund T, Ylikoski M, et al. Accuracy of pedicle screw insertion with and without computer assistance: a randomised controlled clinical study in 100 consecutive patients. Eur Spine J 2000;9(3):235–40.

30. Sanders WP, Truumees E. Imaging of the postoperative spine. Semin Ultrasound CT MR 2004;25(6):523–35. http://dx.doi.org/10.1053/j.sult.2004.09.007.

31. Annertz M, Jönsson B, Strömqvist B, et al. Serial MRI in the early postoperative period after lumbar discectomy. Neuroradiology 1995;37(3):177–82.

32. Van Goethem JW, Van de Kelft E, Biltjes IG, et al. MRI after successful lumbar discectomy. Neuroradiology 1996;38:90–6.

33. Boden SD, Davis DO, Dina TS, et al. Contrast-enhanced MR imaging performed after successful lumbar disk surgery: prospective study. Radiology 1992;182(1):59–64.

34. Ross JS, Masaryk TJ, Modic MT, et al. Lumbar spine: postoperative assessment with surface-coil MR imaging. Radiology 1987;164(3):851–60.

35. Thakkar RS, Malloy JP, Thakkar SC, et al. Imaging the postoperative spine. Radiol Clin North Am 2012;50(4):731–47. http://dx.doi.org/10.1016/j.rcl.2012.04.006.

36. Sethi A, Craig J, Bartol S, et al. Radiographic and CT evaluation of recombinant human bone morphogenetic protein-2-assisted spinal interbody fusion. Am J Roentgenol 2011;197(1):W128–33. http://dx.doi.org/10.2214/AJR.10.5484.

37. Young PM, Berquist TH, Bancroft LW, et al. Complications of spinal instrumentation. Radiographics 2007;27(3):775–89. http://dx.doi.org/10.1148/rg.273065055.

38. Lonstein JE, Denis F, Perra JH, et al. Complications associated with pedicle screws. J Bone Joint Surg Am 1999;81(11):1519–28.

39. Allouni AK, Davis W, Mankad K, et al. Modern spinal instrumentation. Part 2: Multimodality imaging approach for assessment of complications. Clin Radiol 2013;68(1):75–81. http://dx.doi.org/10.1016/j.crad.2012.05.002.

40. Grane P. The postoperative lumbar spine. A radiological investigation of the lumbar spine after discectomy using MR imaging and CT. Acta Radiol Suppl 1998;414:1–23.

41. Bundschuh CV, Stein L, Slusser JH, et al. Distinguishing between scar and recurrent herniated disk in postoperative patients: value of contrast-enhanced CT and MR imaging. AJNR Am J Neuroradiol 1990;11(5):949–58.

42. Ross JS. Magnetic resonance imaging of the postoperative spine. Semin Musculoskelet Radiol 2000;4(3):281–91.

43. Luetmer PH, Mokri B. Dynamic CT myelography: a technique for localizing high-flow spinal cerebrospinal fluid leaks. AJNR Am J Neuroradiol 2003;24(8):1711–4.

44. Kim DH, Rosenblum JK, Panghaal VS, et al. Differentiating neoplastic from nonneoplastic processes in the anterior extradural space. Radiology 2011;260(3):825–30. http://dx.doi.org/10.1148/radiol.11102287.

45. Yi S, Yoon DH, Kim KN, et al. Postoperative spinal epidural hematoma: risk factor and clinical outcome. Yonsei Med J 2006;47(3):326–32.

46. Scavarda D, Peruzzi P, Bazin A, et al. Postoperative spinal extradural hematomas. 14 cases. Neurochirurgie 1997;43(4):220 [in French].

47. Lawton MT, Porter RW, Heiserman JE, et al. Surgical management of spinal epidural hematoma: relationship between surgical timing and neurological outcome. J Neurosurg 1995;83(1):1–7. http://dx.doi.org/10.3171/jns.1995.83.1.0001.

48. Uribe J, Moza K, Jimenez O, et al. Delayed postoperative spinal epidural hematomas. Spine J 2003; 3(2):125–9.

49. Nawashiro H, Higo R. Contrast enhancement of a hyperacute spontaneous spinal epidural hematoma. AJNR Am J Neuroradiol 2001;22(7):1445.

50. Brodsky AE, Kovalsky ES, Khalil MA. Correlation of radiologic assessment of lumbar spine fusions with surgical exploration. Spine 1991;16(Suppl 6): S261–5.

51. Laasonen EM, Soini J. Low-back pain after lumbar fusion. Surgical and computed tomographic analysis. Spine 1989;14(2):210–3.

52. Goldstein C, Drew B. When is a spine fused? Injury 2011;42(3):306–13. http://dx.doi.org/10.1016/j.injury.2010.11.041.

53. Ho JM, Ben-Galim PJ, Weiner BK, et al. Toward the establishment of optimal computed tomographic parameters for the assessment of lumbar spinal fusion. Spine J 2011;11(7):636–40. http://dx.doi.org/10.1016/j.spinee.2011.04.027.

54. Laoutliev B, Havsteen I, Bech BH, et al. Interobserver agreement in fusion status assessment after instrumental desis of the lower lumbar spine using 64-slice multidetector computed tomography: impact of observer experience. Eur Spine J 2012; 21(10):2085–90. http://dx.doi.org/10.1007/s00586-012-2192-4.

55. Cunningham BW, Kanayama M, Parker LM, et al. Osteogenic protein versus autologous interbody arthrodesis in the sheep thoracic spine. A comparative endoscopic study using the Bagby and Kuslich interbody fusion device. Spine 1999;24(6): 509–18.

56. Kuslich SD, Ulstrom CL, Griffith SL, et al. The Bagby and Kuslich method of lumbar interbody fusion. History, techniques, and 2-year follow-up results of a United States prospective, multicenter trial. Spine 1998;23(11):1267–78. http://dx.doi.org/10.1103/PhysRevD.15.2752 [discussion: 1279].

57. Cook SD, Patron LP, Christakis PM, et al. Comparison of methods for determining the presence and extent of anterior lumbar interbody fusion. Spine 2004;29(10):1118–23.

58. Santos ER, Goss DG, Morcom RK, et al. Radiologic assessment of interbody fusion using carbon fiber cages. Spine 2003;28(10):997–1001. http://dx.doi.org/10.1097/01.BRS.0000061988.93175.74.

59. Shah RR, Mohammed S, Saifuddin A, et al. Comparison of plain radiographs with CT scan to evaluate interbody fusion following the use of titanium interbody cages and transpedicular instrumentation. Eur Spine J 2003;12(4):378–85. http://dx.doi.org/10.1007/s00586-002-0517-4.

60. Herzog RJ, Marcotte PJ. Assessment of spinal fusion. Critical evaluation of imaging techniques. Spine 1996;21(9):1114–8.

61. Cizek GR, Boyd LM. Imaging pitfalls of interbody spinal implants. Spine 2000;25(20):2633–6.

62. Sennst DA, Kachelriess M, Leidecker C, et al. An extensible software-based platform for reconstruction and evaluation of CT images. Radiographics 2004;24(2):601–13. http://dx.doi.org/10.1148/rg.242035119.

63. Marchi L, Abdala N, Oliveira L, et al. Radiographic and clinical evaluation of cage subsidence after stand-alone lateral interbody fusion. J Neurosurg Spine 2013;19(1):110–8. http://dx.doi.org/10.3171/2013.4.SPINE12319.

64. Mannion RJ, Nowitzke AM, Wood MJ. Promoting fusion in minimally invasive lumbar Interbody stabilization with low-dose bone morphogenic protein-2—but what is the cost? Spine J 2011;11(6):527–33. http://dx.doi.org/10.1016/j.spinee.2010.07.005.

65. Molinari RW, Bridwell KH, Klepps SJ, et al. Minimum 5-year follow-up of anterior column structural allografts in the thoracic and lumbar spine. Spine 1999;24(10):967–72.

66. Tan GH, Goss BG, Thorpe PJ, et al. CT-based classification of long spinal allograft fusion. Eur Spine J 2007;16(11):1875–81. http://dx.doi.org/10.1007/s00586-007-0376-0.

67. Togawa D, Bauer TW, Lieberman IH, et al. Histologic evaluation of human vertebral bodies after vertebral augmentation with polymethyl methacrylate. Spine 2003;28(14):1521–7.

68. Nakashima H, Yukawa Y, Ito K, et al. Extension CT scan: its suitability for assessing fusion after posterior lumbar interbody fusion. Eur Spine J 2011; 20(9):1496–502. http://dx.doi.org/10.1007/s00586-011-1739-0.

69. Carreon LY, Glassman SD, Schwender JD, et al. Reliability and accuracy of fine-cut computed tomography scans to determine the status of anterior interbody fusions with metallic cages. Spine J 2008;8(6):998–1002. http://dx.doi.org/10.1016/j.spinee.2007.12.004.

70. Katayama Y, Matsuyama Y, Yoshihara H, et al. Clinical and radiographic outcomes of posterolateral lumbar spine fusion in humans using recombinant human bone morphogenetic protein-2: an average five-year follow-up study. Int Orthop 2008;33(4):1061–7. http://dx.doi.org/10.1007/s00264-008-0600-5.

71. Lee P, Fessler RG. Perioperative and postoperative complications of single-level minimally invasive transforaminal lumbar interbody fusion in elderly adults. J Clin Neurosci 2012;19(1):111–4. http://dx.doi.org/10.1016/j.jocn.2011.09.005.

72. Hayeri M, Tehranzadeh J. Diagnostic imaging of spinal fusion and complications. Appl Radiol 2009;38:14–28.

73. Filip M, Linzer P, Strnad J. Development and clinical evaluation of bioactive implant for interbody fusion in the treatment of degenerative lumbar

spine disease. In: Sakai Y, editor. Low back pain pathogenesis and treatment. InTech; 2012. p. 201.

74. Glassman S, Gornet MF, Branch C, et al. Short form 36 and oswestry disability index outcomes after lumbar spine fusion: a multicenter experience. Spine J 2006;6(1):21–6. http://dx.doi.org/10.1016/j.spinee.2005.05.072.

75. Robinson Y, Michaëlsson K, Sandén B. Instrumentation in lumbar fusion improves back pain but not quality of life 2 years after surgery. Acta Orthop 2013;84(1):7–11. http://dx.doi.org/10.3109/17453674.2013.771300.

76. Hussain A, Erdek M. Interventional pain management for failed back surgery syndrome. Pain Pract 2014; 14:64–78. http://dx.doi.org/10.1111/papr.12035.

77. Barzouhi el A, Vleggeert-Lankamp CL, Lycklama à Nijeholt GJ, et al. Magnetic resonance imaging in follow-up assessment of sciatica. N Engl J Med 2013;368(11):999–1007. http://dx.doi.org/10.1056/NEJMoa1209250.

78. Cho W, Shimer AL, Shen FH. Complications associated with posterior lumbar surgery. Seminars in Spine Surgery 2011;23(2):101–13. http://dx.doi.org/10.1053/j.semss.2010.12.013.

79. Lee MJ, Kim S, Lee SA, et al. Overcoming artifacts from metallic orthopedic implants at high-field-strength MR imaging and multi-detector CT. Radiographics 2007;27(3):791–803. http://dx.doi.org/10.1148/rg.273065087.

80. Fogel GR, Toohey JS, Neidre A, et al. Fusion assessment of posterior lumbar interbody fusion using radiolucent cages: X-ray films and helical computed tomography scans compared with surgical exploration of fusion. Spine J 2008;8(4):570–7. http://dx.doi.org/10.1016/j.spinee.2007.03.013.

81. Waguespack A, Schofferman J, Slosar P, et al. Etiology of long-term failures of lumbar spine surgery. Pain Med 2002;3(1):18–22. http://dx.doi.org/10.1046/j.1526-4637.2002.02007.x.

82. Douglas-Akinwande AC, Buckwalter KA, Rydberg J, et al. Multichannel CT: evaluating the spine in post-operative patients with orthopedic hardware1. Radiographics 2006;26(Suppl 1):S97–110. http://dx.doi.org/10.1148/rg.26si065512.

83. Delamarter RB, Ross JS, Masaryk TJ, et al. Diagnosis of lumbar arachnoiditis by magnetic resonance imaging. Spine 1990;15(4):304–10.

84. Hawk MW, Kim KD. Review of spinal pseudomeningoceles and cerebrospinal fluid fistulas. Neurosurg Focus 2000;9(1):e5.

85. Teplick JG, Peyster RG, Teplick SK, et al. CT identification of postlaminectomy pseudomeningocele. AJR Am J Roentgenol 1983;140(6):1203–6.

86. Etebar S, Cahill DW. Risk factors for adjacent-segment failure following lumbar fixation with rigid instrumentation for degenerative instability. J Neurosurg 1999;90(Suppl 2):163–9.

87. Park P, Garton HJ, Gala VC, et al. Adjacent segment disease after lumbar or lumbosacral fusion: review of the literature. Spine 2004;29(17): 1938–44.

88. Fujibayashi S, Takemoto M, Izeki M, et al. Does the formation of vertebral endplate cysts predict nonunion after lumbar interbody fusion? Spine 2012;37(19):E1197–202. http://dx.doi.org/10.1097/BRS.0b013e31825d26d7.

Motion Preservation Surgery in the Spine

Ryan Murtagh, MD, MBA[a],*, Antonio E. Castellvi, MD[†,b]

KEYWORDS

• Spine • Motion preservation • Total disc replacement

KEY POINTS

- The primary goal of motion preservation surgery is to maintain normal or near normal motion in an attempt to prevent adverse outcomes commonly seen with conventional spinal fusion, most notably the development of adjacent-level degenerative disc disease.
- There are several different approaches developed to preserve motion in the lumbar spine, including total disc replacement, partial disc (nucleus) replacement, interspinous spacers, dynamic stabilization devices, and total facet replacement devices.
- The design of lumbar total disc replacement devices varies greatly. Commonly seen complications include subsidence, migration, fracture, heterotopic ossification, and even adjacent-segment degeneration.
- Cervical motion preservation surgery primarily consists of total disc replacement. The devices are created using a similar rationale but are unique in design relative to their lumbar counterparts.

Discectomy and spinal fusion is considered the gold standard for the treatment of symptomatic degenerative disc disease.[1,2] Though often effective in the short term, it is not without significant morbidity. Perhaps one of the most commonly recognized adverse outcomes of spinal fusion is the development of degenerative disc disease at the level(s) adjacent to a spinal fusion procedure.

Motion preservation surgery in the spine, while not a novel concept, has seen a significant increase in use during the last decade, particularly with respect to disc arthroplasty (total disc replacement) devices in the cervical and lumbar spine. The goal of motion preservation surgery, in general, is to closely replicate normal or near normal biomechanics in an effort to restore patient mobility and minimize the development of clinically significant adjacent-segment disc disease.[1]

Although relatively new in the spine, motion preservation surgery is a well-established surgical technique in the appendicular skeleton, and the benefits of hip and knee joint replacement, among

others, are clearly recognized. The spinal motion segment, or functional spinal unit, is more complex than the appendicular joints. The functional spinal unit is effectively composed of 3 joints: the disc space and 2 facet joints. As such, the relatively simple principles of replacing a single joint in the appendicular skeleton are not applicable, and the complex interaction among these 3 articulating components must be taken into consideration before surgical intervention. As a result, there is a vast array of devices available in spinal motion preservation surgery, particularly in the lumbar spine. In the lumbar spine, devices can be loosely grouped into anterior and posterior motion-preserving devices. Cervical motion preservation surgery presents with more limited options and mainly consists of total disc replacement (TDR).

In the lumbar spine, anterior motion preservation devices, or devices intended to replicate the normal motion of the disc space, include TDR and partial disc (nucleus) replacement. TDR is a well-established surgical technique with a

† Deceased.
a University of South Florida, 2700 University Square Drive, Tampa, FL 33612, USA; b Orthopaedic Research and Education, Florida Orthopaedic Institute, Tampa, FL 33637, USA
* Corresponding author.
E-mail address: rmurtagh13@gmail.com

Neuroimag Clin N Am 24 (2014) 287–294
http://dx.doi.org/10.1016/j.nic.2014.01.008

neuroimaging.theclinics.com

multitude of devices available. Although cervical and lumbar TDR procedures are designed with the same rationale (ie, replace the abnormal disc while restoring near normal biomechanics), the devices are distinctly unique in design and, in many cases, the frequency and specific type of postoperative complications. In partial disc replacement, the diseased nucleus pulposus is replaced or augmented with an injectable or preformed device (Fig. 1). The complex, preformed partial disc replacement devices require relatively invasive surgery while some of the injectable materials can be administered through a minimally invasive percutaneous approach. The goal of partial disc replacement is to increase disc space height and maintain near normal motion in an attempt to minimize the development of adjacent-segment disease.

There are several types of posterior motion preservation devices, including interspinous spacers, dynamic stabilization screws and rods, and total facet replacement. Interspinous spacers (Fig. 2) are devices placed between the spinous processes of adjacent levels. The primary goal of this procedure is to increase disc space height in an attempt to decrease canal stenosis and relieve neurogenic claudication. This procedure is relatively noninvasive, particularly in comparison with

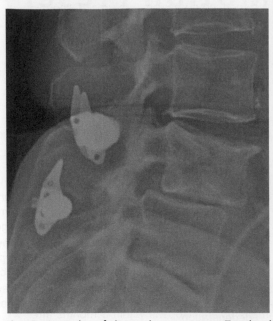

Fig. 2. Example of interspinous spacer. Two-level X-stop (Kyphon, Sunnyvale, CA) interspinous spacer implanted at L3-L4 and L4-L5 levels.

TDR, and typically does not preclude other types of surgery in the event of failure. Dynamic stabilization devices are similar to traditional pedicle screw-and-rod constructs in many aspects. These devices, however, are not rigid, allowing for a small amount of movement through mobile portions of the screws or rods. The goal of these devices is to stabilize the spine while simultaneously allowing for a small amount of motion. Facet replacement is a relatively invasive procedure whereby a laminectomy and bilateral facetectomy is performed and a prosthetic facet device implanted (Fig. 3). The goal of facet replacement is to relieve canal and foraminal stenosis while maintaining some degree of motion at the affected level.

Motion preservation surgery of the spine is a complex, constantly evolving field. While the general principles of spinal motion preservation surgery remain relatively constant, many of the specific devices in use as recently as 2 to 3 years ago are no longer clinically available, having failed clinical trials, lost funding, or been simply deemed ineffective. New devices enter clinical trials every year. Given the dynamic nature of this field, the remainder of this article emphasizes TDR. TDR is the most commonly performed of the motion-preserving surgeries. There are many established cervical and lumbar TDR devices, several of which have been approved by the Food and Drug Administration (FDA) for clinical use in the United States. As a result, there are many large randomized

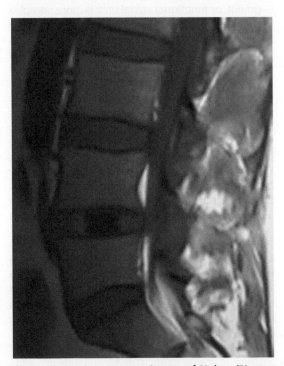

Fig. 1. Magnetic resonance image of Nubac (Pioneer Surgical Technology, Marquette, MI). The device consists of 2 polyetherether ketone (PEEK) endplates with a ball-and-socket articulation. (*Courtesy of* Chip Bao, PhD.)

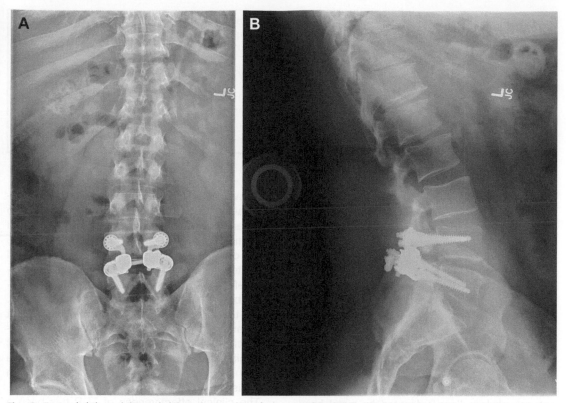

Fig. 3. Frontal (*A*) and lateral (*B*) radiographs of the Acadia (Facet Solutions, Hopkinton, MA) total facet replacement.

controlled trials documenting the surgeries and comparing TDR with conventional fusion.

LUMBAR TOTAL DISC REPLACEMENT

Lumbar TDR devices vary widely in shape and composition. Some, like the Charité device (DePuy Spine, Raynham, MA), have a 3-component design with metal endplates and a polyethylene liner. Others, like the FlexiCore device (Stryker Spine, Summit, NJ) are a 2-part, metal-only design that uses a ball-and-socket type articulation between the endplates. Some of the endplates of these devices are relatively flat and must use small "teeth" along the endplates to maintain purchase with the adjacent vertebral body; this is seen, for example, in the Charité device (**Fig. 4**). Others, like the ProDisc-L device (Synthes Spine USA Products LLC, West Chester, PA), use large, vertical endplate keels to maintain purchase.

Most of these devices require an invasive anterior approach. The exception is NuVasive's XL TDR (Nuvasive Manufacturing LLC, Fairborn, OH), which is implanted indirectly through a far-lateral approach (**Fig. 5**). TDR surgeries in general are relatively invasive, and revision is often difficult in the event of hardware failure.

From an imaging standpoint it is important for the radiologist to be aware of the potential complications of TDR. In the immediate postoperative setting the radiologist should be able to identify surgical complications related to the approach. Most of these are implanted from an anterior approach, and complications including inadvertent peritoneal entry and vascular injury, though rare, can occur in the postoperative setting. In the case of the Nuvasive device a far-lateral approach is used, and the radiologist should search for retroperitoneal or inadvertent peritoneal complications related to the lateral approach. Other early complications include fracture of the vertebral body/endplates from aggressive implantation, and this should be investigated in the symptomatic postoperative patient (**Table 1**).

Chronic complications include subsidence, migration, and the development of heterotopic ossification and adjacent-level disease. Subsidence refers to the slow settling of the device into the endplates. Most of the surface area of the device will contact the softer bone located central to the outer ring apophysis. Subsidence is particularly prevalent in cases where implant is undersized and the footplate of the device is

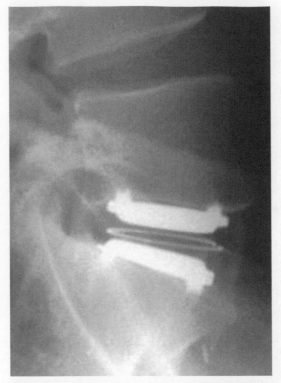

Fig. 4. Charité total disc replacement (TDR). Radiolucent polyethylene liner is denoted by metal band. Note small "teeth" along endplates to maintain purchase.

significantly smaller than the surface area of the adjacent vertebral body. Migration is relatively uncommon but can, like subsidence, occur in the setting of undersized devices. In cases of migration, the compressive forces of the vertebral bodies do not have sufficient strength to contain

Table 1
Complications associated with lumbar total disc replacement

Early	Hemorrhage, vascular injury, infection, peritoneal entry, vertebral fracture
Late	Subsidence of implant, implant migration, heterotopic ossification, adjacent-level degenerative disc disease

the device within the disc space. Migration is typically along the operative path, and migration into the paraspinal soft tissues or psoas muscle can potentially occur if a far-lateral approach is used. Many devices use endplate keels (**Fig. 6**) or small teeth to minimize migration. Heterotopic ossification refers to the gradual development of heterotopic bone along the periphery of the interspace. Often this is asymptomatic, and is only significant from an imaging standpoint. With significant heterotopic ossification there can, in some cases, be limitation of the range of motion, and in severe cases there can even be bridging bone with autofusion.[3]

The clinical effectiveness of TDR has been a source of debate and extensive study. TDR is a relatively new concept and, while some devices have been in place for a decade or more, most well-designed randomized controlled studies are still in the earlier stages. Recent trials have failed to show superiority of TDR over fusion. A meta-analysis of 6 randomized controlled trials consisting of 1603 patients reviewed the safety and efficacy of lumbar TDR in comparison with lumbar fusion. Although there was significant safety and efficacy of TDR versus fusion, TDR was not be shown to be superior to fusion.[4]

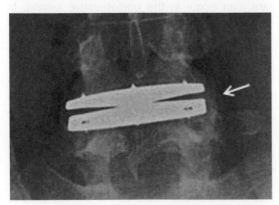

Fig. 5. Nuvasive XL TDR. The device is implanted through an indirect far-lateral approach, similar to that used with extreme lateral lumbar interbody fusion technique. Note heterotopic ossification along the left lateral aspect of the device (*arrow*).

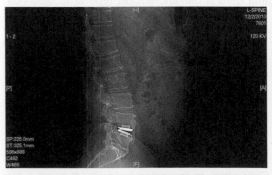

Fig. 6. Scout computed tomography image of the lumbar spine with ProDisc at L4-L5 showing bridging heterotopic ossification. Note the large vertical keel of the ProDisc device designed to prevent migration.

Another meta-analysis of 837 patients enrolled in 5 randomized controlled trials compared the effectiveness and safety of lumbar TDR versus fusion.[5,6] In this review the function, pain level, and patient satisfaction status between the 2 groups was not significantly different at 5 years. The complication and reoperation rates were also similar at 5 years. The investigators concluded that lumbar TDR was not significantly superior to lumbar fusion for the treatment of lumbar degenerative disc disease.[5]

The primary justification for lumbar TDR and motion preservation surgery is to prevent or minimize the development of adjacent-level disease (ALD) and abnormality.[1,3] In addition to debating the clinical efficacy of TDR, there has been significant debate about the rate and even the significance of ALD and abnormality as regards fusion versus TDR. One theory for the development of ALD is that the altered mechanics of traditional lumbar fusion leads to abnormal stress on the adjacent motion segment and, in turn, promotes degeneration. This situation would justify the use of motion preservation surgery. Others argue that the development of ALD is simply part of the normal degenerative cascade. In 2012, Wang and colleagues[7] performed a literature review in an effort to establish rates of ALD in lumbar TDR in comparison with fusion. The review, which included articles from 1990 through 2012, found "moderate evidence" that clinically significant ALD was almost 6 times more likely to occur with fusion than with TDR. Specifically, the investigators found that the pooled risk of clinically significant ALD requiring surgical intervention was 1.2% in TDR and 7.0% in fusion. Another study assessed 5-year results for radiographically demonstrated ALD in patients treated with ProDisc-L versus circumferential fusion. In this review, the patients treated with circumferential fusion were greater than 3 times more likely to demonstrate findings of ALD (radiographically identified as loss of disc space height, osteophytosis, endplate sclerosis, or spondylolisthesis).[8]

CERVICAL TOTAL DISC REPLACEMENT

The principles of cervical TDR are similar to those in lumbar TDR. In cervical TDR there is removal of the diseased disc and implantation of the arthroplasty device. In addition to neural decompression, the goal is to restore normal or near normal motion so as to minimize ALD. ALD has been shown to occur with increased frequency at the levels adjacent to anterior cervical discectomy and fusion (ACDF) in several studies. In one study,

up to 25% of patients with ACDF experienced symptomatic ALD.[9] Other post-ACDF problems potentially alleviated by cervical TDR include stiffness, nonunion, hardware failure, and dysphagia.[10] At present there are 3 devices with FDA approval in the United States but only 2 that are available for commercial use. The 2 devices approved for commercial use are the ProDisc-C (Synthes Spine USA) and Prestige ST (Medtronic, Memphis, TN).

The devices, like lumbar TDR, vary greatly in design. The Bryan Cervical Disc System device (Medtronic) consists of 2 titanium endplates with a polyurethane core. The Prestige device (Fig. 7) consists of 2 stainless-steel blade-shaped endplates that are anchored to the vertebral bodies by anterior screws. Other devices, such as the Kineflex-C (Spinal Motion LLC, Mountain View, CA) are composed of cobalt-chromium-molybdenum alloy and use designs that more closely parallel those of their lumbar counterparts. Some devices, such as the ProDisc-C, use vertical keels for stabilization, whereas others use teeth for endplate purchase. The Discover TDR device (Depuy Spine, Inc, Raynham, MA) consists of 2 radiopaque titanium endplates and a radiolucent ultra–high molecular weight polyethylene core (Fig. 8).

Complications of cervical TDR are similar to those for the lumbar spine and include fracture, subsidence, migration, heterotopic ossification, and hardware failure or loosening. Subsidence,

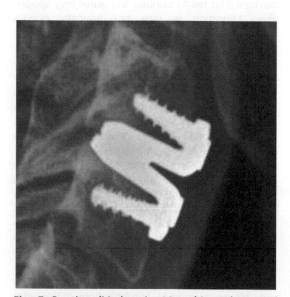

Fig. 7. Prestige (Medtronic, Memphis, TN) cervical TDR. The device is composed of stainless steel and consists of 2 articulating metal endplates held in place by screws at the adjacent vertebral body levels.

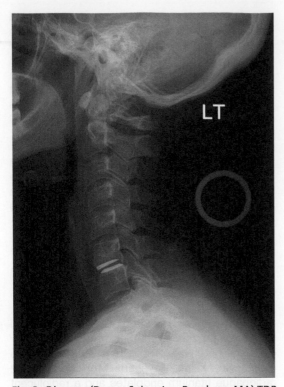

Fig. 8. Discover (Depuy Spine, Inc, Raynham, MA) TDR device.

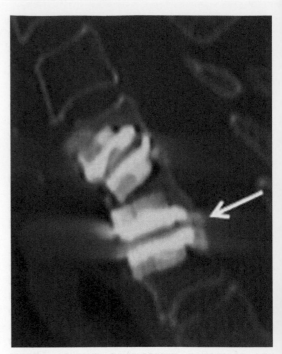

Fig. 9. Two-level cervical TDR using ProDisc-C (r) (Synthes Spine, West Chester, PA). There is subsidence of both devices, to the point that they are nearly touching. In addition, there is heterotopic ossification seen at both levels, more so along the posterior aspect of the more caudal device (*arrow*).

as in lumbar TDR, is a gradual process whereby the device settles into the adjacent vertebral body (**Fig. 9**). It is often seen with undersized devices that fail to contact the outer ring apophysis. Migration is rare but typically occurs anteriorly, along the operative approach (**Fig. 10**). Heterotopic ossification is seen with relative frequency in the cervical spine, such frequency varying according to the device. In one study the frequency of heterotopic ossification in 3 devices was 40%. More specifically, it was seen in 21% of Bryan devices, 52.5% of the Mobi-C devices, and 71.4% of ProDisc-C devices.[11] There was also an increased prevalence of heterotopic ossification in men compared with women (47.6% vs 29.2%). In another study that reviewed the ProDisc-C device, 45% of devices demonstrated grade III (extends into disc space and limits motion) heterotopic ossification and 18% demonstrated grade IV (bridges disc space and results in fusion) heterotopic ossification.[12] A third study found heterotopic ossification in 50% of Bryan implants, but only 4% of these were grade III and only 2% were grade IV. The limitations of this latter study were a relatively small sample size (36 patients) and a relatively short follow-up period (only 12 months).[13]

Like lumbar TDR, there are several trials in progress. Recently, the 5-year results of cervical TDR with ProDisc-C versus ACDF were published. Both groups showed clinically significant improvement at both 2 and 5 years versus baseline. At 5 years the ProDisc-C group had statistically significantly less severe and less frequent neck pain relative to the ACDF group. There were no reported device failures or implant migration. In addition, the ProDisc-C group had a statistically significantly lower rate of reoperation relative to ACDF (2.9% vs 11.3%).[10] In similar fashion, a review of reoperation rates in a series of 6 FDA Investigational Device Exemption studies using cervical TDR in comparison with ACDF found a significantly decreased reoperation rate in the TDR group when compared with the ACDF group (8.3% vs 21.2%). Specifically, the reoperation rate for ALD was 4.8% in the TDR group versus 13.5% in the ACDF group. There was a significantly longer survival period before reoperation in the TDR group than in ACDF group.[14] A meta-analysis of 13 reports from 10 randomized controlled trials involving 2227 patients showed better function, less frequent reoperation, and lower major complication rates for TDR patients

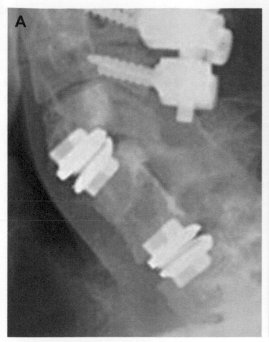
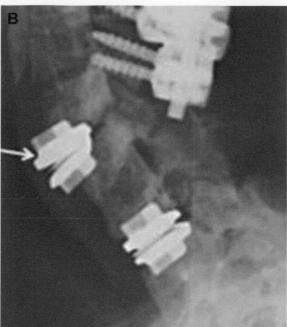

Fig. 10. Migration immediately postoperatively (*A*) and 4 months after surgery (*B*) after 2-level cervical TDR using ProDisc-C (r) (Synthes Spine, West Chester, PA). At 4-month follow-up, the more cranial device was noted to have migrated anteriorly (*arrow*).

in comparison with patients undergoing fusion procedures. This analysis, however, did not find a significant difference in the rate of reoperation attributable to adjacent-segment degeneration.[15] Finally, a systematic review of the literature found no significant difference in the frequency of radiographic or clinically significant adjacent-segment abnormality in short-term to mid-term follow-up of patients treated with TDR rather than ACDF.[16]

DEDICATION

Dr Antonio Castellvi, or "Doc" as he is affectionately known by peers, friends and family, passed away on February 8th, 2014 at the age of 61. Dr Castellvi was a leader in the field of spine surgery. He was head of the Spine Fellowship at the University of South Florida and director of the biomechanics lab at the Foundation for Orthopedic Education and Research. Dr Castellvi presented and moderated at multiple meetings at the national and international level but will perhaps most fondly be remembered for his popular annual meeting Current Solutions in Spine Surgery in Duck Key, FL. Dr Castellvi was widely respected by his peers and patients and he will be dearly missed.

REFERENCES

1. Errico TJ. Why a mechanical disc? Spine J 2004; 4(Suppl 6):151S–7S.

2. Lemaire JP, Carrier H, Sariali el-H, et al. Clinical and radiological outcomes with the Charité artificial disc: a 10-year minimum follow-up. J Spinal Disord Tech 2005;18(4):353–9 [Published correction appears in J Spinal Disord Tech 2006; 19(1):76.].

3. Murtagh RD, Quencer RM, Castellvi AE, et al. New techniques in lumbar spinal instrumentation: what the radiologist needs to know. Radiology 2011;260: 317–30.

4. Wei J, Song Y, Sun L, et al. Comparison of artificial total disc replacement versus fusion for lumbar degenerative disc disease: a meta-analysis of randomized controlled trials. Int Orthop 2013;37: 1315–25.

5. Yajun W, Yue Z, Hiuxin H. A meta-analysis of artificial total disc replacement versus fusion for lumbar degenerative disc disease. Eur Spine J 2010;19: 1250–61.

6. Murtagh RD, Quencer RM, Cohen DS, et al. Normal and abnormal imaging findings in lumbar total disk replacement: devices and complications. Radiographics 2009;29(1):105–18.

7. Wang JC, Arnold PM, Hermsmeyer JT, et al. Do lumbar motion preserving devices reduce the risk of adjacent segment pathology compared with fusion surgery? Spine 2012;37(22S):S133–43.

8. Ziegler JE, Glenn J, Delamarter RB. Five-year adjacent-level degenerative changes in patients with single-level disease treated using lumbar total

disc replacement with ProDisc-L versus circumferential fusion. J Neurosurg Spine 2012;17(6):504–11.

9. Azmi H, Schlenk R. Surgery for post arthrodesis adjacent-cervical segment degeneration. Neurosurg Focus 2003;15:E6.

10. Zigler JE, Delamarter R, Murrey D, et al. ProDisc-C and anterior cervical discectomy and fusion as surgical treatment for single-level cervical symptomatic degenerative disc disease. Spine 2013;38(3):203–9.

11. Yi S, Shin DA, Kim KN. The predisposing factors for the heterotopic ossification after cervical artificial total disc replacement. Spine J 2013;13:1048–54.

12. Suchomel P, Jurak L, Benes V, et al. Clinical results and development of heterotopic ossification in total cervical disc replacement during a 4-year follow-up. Eur Spine J 2010;19(2):307–15.

13. Tu TH, Wu JC, Wang WC, et al. Heterotopic ossification after cervical total disc replacement: determination by CT and effects on clinical outcomes. J Neurosurg Spine 2011;14(4):457–65.

14. Blumenthal SL, Ohnmeiss DD, Guyer R, et al. Reoperations in cervical total disc replacement compared with anterior cervical fusion. Spine 2013;38:1177–82.

15. Yin S, Yu X, Zhou S, et al. Is cervical disc arthroplasty superior to fusion for treatment of symptomatic cervical disc disease? A meta-analysis. Clin Orthop Relat Res 2013;471:1904–19.

16. Harrod CC, Hillibrand AS, Fischer DJ, et al. Adjacent segment pathology following cervical motion-sparing procedures or devices compared with fusion surgery. Spine 2012;37(22S):S96–112.

The Postoperative Spine
What the Spine Surgeon Needs to Know

Roi M. Bittane, MD[a],*, Alexandre B. de Moura, MD[b],
Ruby J. Lien, MD[a]

KEYWORDS

- Postoperative spine • Spinal surgery • Imaging • Complications

KEY POINTS

- Imaging plays a crucial role in the evaluation of the postoperative spine and significantly influences subsequent clinical management of the patient.
- A basic understanding of spine surgical procedures is essential to the proper evaluation of the postoperative spine.
- Imaging allows for excellent delineation of both normal and abnormal findings in the postoperative spine. It is critically important to learn to differentiate normal findings from abnormal findings to be of clinical use.
- This article provides the radiologist the basic tools required to evaluate the manifestations and complications of spine surgery properly on imaging studies.

INTRODUCTION

Radiologists are often tasked with the interpretation of postoperative spine imaging, the goal being to assist the surgeon in the continued clinical management of the patient. Imaging evaluation of the postoperative spine is complex and requires a detailed understanding of the initial spinal pathologic condition, the surgical procedure performed, the clinical presentation of the patient, and the time interval from the surgery to the imaging study. Imaging plays a crucial role in the assessment of the postoperative spine. It is essential in identifying the location and integrity of surgical implants, in evaluating the success of decompression procedures, in delineating fusion status, and in identifying postoperative complications.

This article provides the reader with the fundamental tools required to evaluate postoperative spine imaging and create effective reports to guide the spine surgeon in patient management. It addresses the basic surgical procedures and hardware commonly used in modern spine surgery. In addition, proper evaluation of the spine following these procedures is delineated, with an emphasis on the information most critical to the treating physician. Finally, general postsurgical complications pertaining to the spine are also reviewed.

SURGICAL TECHNIQUES

A thorough evaluation of the postoperative spine begins with a clear understanding of the patient's presentation history and surgical procedure performed.

Spine surgeries can be divided into 3 main categories of procedures,[1–4] as listed in **Box 1**.

This section reviews some of the more common surgical techniques as well as the hardware involved in these procedures.

Decompressive Procedures

The decompressive procedures are most often performed to remove herniated disc material encroaching on the neural elements or to relieve

[a] Department of Radiology, Winthrop University Hospital, Mineola, NY 11501, USA; [b] NYU School Of Medicine, New York, NY 10016, USA
* Corresponding author.
E-mail address: Rbittane@winthrop.org

Neuroimag Clin N Am 24 (2014) 295–303
http://dx.doi.org/10.1016/j.nic.2014.01.006
1052-5149/14/$ – see front matter © 2014 Elsevier Inc. All rights reserved.

a segment of spinal stenosis. These procedures are most often performed from a posterior midline approach at the level of the lumbar spine, which provides optimal access to the posterior elements, spinal canal, and the intervertebral disc. There are 3 typical decompressive techniques, laminotomy, laminectomy, and laminectomy with facetectomy.[1,4]

Laminotomy involves only partial resection of the inferior portion of the cephalic lamina and, if necessary, partial resection of the superior portion of the caudal lamina. This procedure often includes a microdiscectomy.[1,4]

Laminectomy involves complete removal of the lamina of the vertebral body and may be unilateral or bilateral. Unilateral laminectomy involves excision of only one lamina of the vertebral body. Bilateral, or total, laminectomy is by definition removal of both laminae as well as the spinous process (**Fig. 1**). In certain cases, portions of the adjacent lamina may also be removed to achieve appropriate decompression or greater exposure of the spinal canal. Laminectomy is often performed to relieve spinal stenosis or when removal of larger disc material is necessary. A notable exception

to this rule occurs at the L5-S1 level, where a discectomy often requires only removal of the ligamentum flavum without bony excision.[1,4]

Laminectomy with complete or partial facetectomy is performed when there is a need to access the neural foramen to relieve nerve root compression. It is important to preserve as much of the lateral facet joint as possible during the decompression so as not to create instability of the spinal segment. Too radical a resection of the facet joint may lead to an iatrogenic spondylolisthesis.[1,4]

Varying degrees of discectomy may be involved in all of the above decompressive procedures.

Stabilization and Fusion Procedures

Spinal stabilization and fusion procedures are performed to address various clinical scenarios including degenerative disc disease, spondylolisthesis, trauma, tumors, and infection. Surgical hardware is used to stabilize the spine, maintain its anatomic alignment, or replace excised components. The specific surgical approach as well as the instrumentation used depends on the clinical setting and the specific pathologic condition to be treated.[1,2,5–7]

Surgical hardware

To gain a better understanding of the specific surgical stabilization techniques, it is important to review the different surgical implants used during spinal stabilization and fusion surgery.

Plates and rods with transpedicular screws Pedicle screws and rods are most often used to form a construct, which stabilizes and/or affixes several vertebral levels (**Fig. 2**). These are routinely used anywhere from the thoracic spine to the sacrum. Rods are attached to screws for multilevel fusion. Each rod can be individually shaped, with cross bars and screws positioned at varying vertebrae so as to provide secure fixation of the spine. Rods and screws are usually attached to the vertebral bodies using transpedicular screws in the thoracic and lumbar spine (lateral mass screws and other screws are used in the cervical spine).[1–3] The screws traverse the pedicle and enter the vertebral body. Although there is no consensus on the optimal length of transpedicular screws, the tip of the screw should not breech the anterior vertebral body cortex, except for the sacrum. The main advantage of using a screw/rod-based construct is that it provides immediate postoperative internal fixation. This fixation allows for maintenance of spinal deformity correction or stabilization of an unstable segment. The application of hardware also ensures an increase in fusion rates.[1–3,5–8]

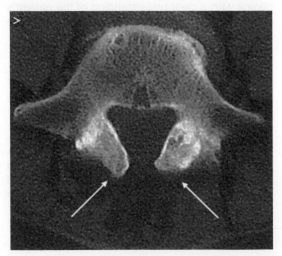

Fig. 1. Axial CT image in bone window algorithm in a 51-year-old female patient after partial bilateral laminectomy (*white arrows*) with removal of the spinous process at the L4-5 intervertebral disc level.

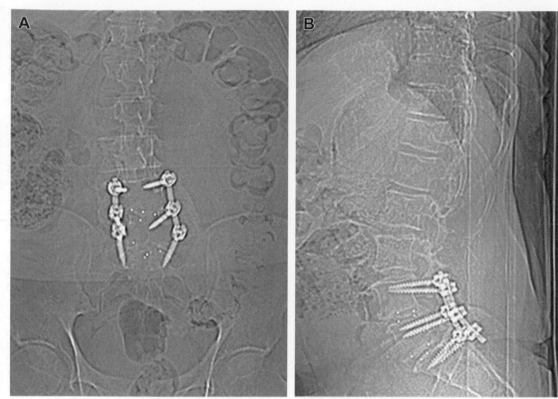

Fig. 2. Typical rod and transpedicular screw construct. Anteroposterior (*A*) and lateral (*B*) images in a 61-year-old male patient after discectomy at the L4-5 and L5-S1 intervertebral levels. There has been subsequent placement of interbody spacers (delineated by punctuate metallic densities) at the L4-5 and L5-S1 intervertebral disc levels with overlying stabilization hardware consisting of bilateral rods and transpedicular screws.

Translaminar or facet screws In cases where the posterior elements are intact, screws may be placed within the lamina or the facet joint.[1–3,8]

Interbody spacers Interbody spacers are solid or openwork structures, often filled with bone graft material, that are placed in the intervertebral disc space after discectomy; they may also be used to replace a resected vertebrae (**Fig. 3**). The spacers' purpose is to promote fusion while maintaining alignment and spinal column support. Spacers are composed of titanium, carbon fiber, polyetheretherketone, or cortical/cortico-cancellous bone graft. Most spacers contain radiopaque markers to allow evaluation of their position. A posterior marker located approximately 2 mm anterior to the posterior edge of the adjacent vertebral body indicates the spacer is in a good position. Important complications involving spacers include retropulsion and cage subsidence.[1,2,8]

Fusion—surgical approaches
Surgical fusion procedures are often categorized based on the direction from which the spine is approached (anterior, posterior, lateral, caudal) as well as on their degree of invasiveness.[1,2,5,6]

A posterior surgical approach is used when decompression is required in addition to fusion.

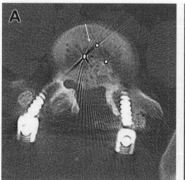
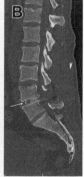

Fig. 3. A 32-year-old male patient after discectomy at the L4-5 intervertebral level. Axial CT image in bone window algorithm (*A*) and sagittal 2D CT reformation in bone window algorithm (*B*) demonstrate optimal placement of an interbody spacer (*white arrows*) at the center of the vertebral body as delineated by radiopaque markers. There is no lateral displacement or retropulsion.

Posterior interbody fusion involves bilateral laminectomy with removal of the intervertebral disc material. Bone graft material and interbody spacers are then packed into the intervertebral space; this is followed by placement of surgical fixation hardware to provide rigid support to the spine until complete bony fusion (see **Fig. 3**).[1,2,5,6]

Transforaminal interbody fusion is a variant of posterior interbody fusion using a posterolateral approach, which leaves the midline structures intact and results in less disruption of the spinal canal. Due to the lateral approach, a total facetectomy is required to access the intervertebral disc space.[1,2]

In cases where there is severe loss of the intervertebral space without the possibility of inserting a spacer, complete posterolateral fusion is performed. In this procedure bone graft material is placed laterally between the transverse processes. Overlying surgical hardware is usually placed to provide additional support to the spinal column.

An anterior surgical approach is used when the patient's pain is discogenic and decompression is not necessary. Anterior interbody fusion involves removal of intervertebral disc material, which is usually replaced by a large interbody cage spacer. This spacer is supplemented by plates placed anteriorly and, if necessary, posterior fixation for added stability. Performing an anterior interbody fusion requires an anterior abdominal incision or a retroperitoneal approach from the flanks as opposed to a posterior (back) midline incision.[1,2,5,6]

Stand-alone interbody fusion addresses the same clinical scenarios as the above-mentioned interbody fusion procedures. However, in this case the interbody cage spacer is directly affixed to the adjacent vertebral bodies using screws, eliminating the need for any additional surgical hardware.[2]

Additional Procedures

Vertebral body replacement (corpectomy)

A vertebral body may require replacement after excision due to tumor, trauma, or infection. The vertebral body replacement hardware often takes the form of an expandable cage filled with bone graft or cement. In most cases, anterior, posterior, or lateral rods/plates with screws are placed for added stability and spinal support.[2,8]

Disc arthroplasty

Disc arthroplasty is performed in cases where pain is thought to originate from disc degeneration without neural involvement. The procedure involves removal of the diseased disc and replacement with an artificial disc composed of a polyethylene core sandwiched between 2 metal plates that attach to the vertebral bodies. The sandwich construct is designed to allow motion and provide cushioning. The main purpose of the procedure is to relieve pain while restoring normal disc space motion. Contraindications to this procedure include facet joint degeneration, prior infection, and spinal segment instability.[2,3]

Dynamic stabilization devices

Dynamic stabilization devices may be of benefit in cases where low back pain is thought to originate from chronic degeneration of the spine. These devices alter the load-bearing and motion of the spine, thereby limiting the strain placed on specific spinous segments and reducing subsequent progressive degeneration. These devices, which are of variable designs and constructs, may be used alone or in conjunction with fusion hardware.[2,4,8]

EVALUATION POSTSURGERY

From the surgeon's perspective, it is imperative to evaluate whether the pathologic condition for which surgery was performed has been treated. As noted earlier, this requires a detailed understanding of the patient's complaints as well as of the findings on preoperative imaging. However, before such evaluation, one must be familiar with and be able to differentiate between expected changes in the postoperative spine and the appearance of true postoperative pathologic condition.

Evaluation Following Decompressive Procedures

Postsurgical changes involving the osseous structures are best appreciated on a computed tomographic (CT) scan (using bone window algorithm). However, for most other purposes, magnetic resonance (MR) imaging is superior because it allows for a better appreciation of the relationship between the osseous structures and the adjacent soft tissues, spinal cord, and exiting nerve roots.[1,9]

Following laminectomy, MR imaging often demonstrates disruption of the margins of the paraspinal muscles as well as edema of the adjacent soft tissues. The laminectomy defect itself is best evaluated on T1-weighted axial images and should correspond to the level of disease on the preoperative imaging study (**Fig. 4**). Note that the dural sac may protrude toward the laminectomy defect; this is within the spectrum of expected postsurgical changes and should not be mistaken for a pseudomeningocele.[1]

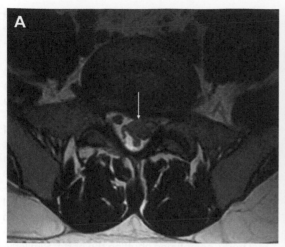
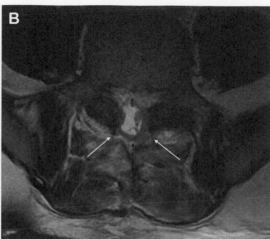

Fig. 4. A 52-year-old female patient after laminectomy at the L5-S1 intervertebral disc level due to an L5-S1 disc herniation. Presurgical (A) T2-weighted axial MR image demonstrates the herniated disc material encroaching on the thecal sac and left S1 nerve root (*white arrow*). Postsurgical T2-weighted axial MR image (B) demonstrates bilateral laminectomy with removal of herniated disc material (*white arrows*). Notice slight posterior protrusion of the dural sac (*black arrow*) as well as mild edema in the posterior lumbar soft tissues and musculature.

When a discectomy has also been performed, it is important to be aware that post-discectomy changes may mimic reherniation. The intraoperative disruption of the annulus fibrosus with resulting edema in the epidural space may indeed mildly efface the thecal sac and mislead the inexperienced radiologist. Additional findings that may be encountered in postoperative patients include contrast enhancement of the vertebral endplates and/or enhancement of the posterior annulus fibrosis.[10–12] These findings often reflect postsurgical aseptic reaction and may be found in completely asymptomatic patients.[1,3,9,13]

A later development that may be observed in the postoperative spine is the formation of epidural fibrosis, which may impinge on the thecal sac and mimic reherniation. To differentiate epidural fibrosis and scarring from a recurrent herniation, it is necessary to administer intravenous contrast. Epidural scar will demonstrate an intermediate signal with irregular margins and heterogeneous early enhancement (Fig. 5). A recurrent disc

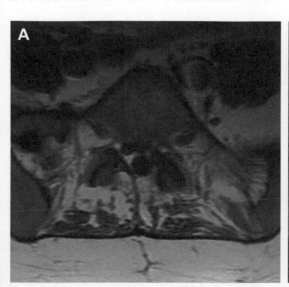
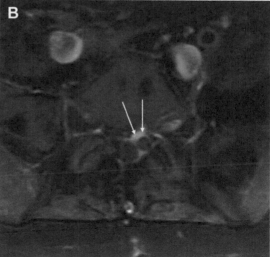

Fig. 5. A 52-year-old female patient with low back pain after left L5-S1 laminectomy and partial discectomy. Non-contrast T1-weighted axial MR image (A) and fat-suppressed contrast-enhanced T1-weighted axial MR image (B) demonstrate enhancing soft tissue in the left anterolateral aspect of the canal (*white arrows*), which surrounds the left S1 nerve root and likely represents scar tissue.

herniation will more often demonstrate a low signal with smooth margins and no early contrast enhancement. In certain situations a recurrent disc herniation may be encased by enhancing scar tissue, making accurate interpretation more complex.[1] In addition, contrast material may diffuse from the epidural scar to the disc material on late contrast-enhanced images. Therefore, it is imperative to obtain images as rapidly as possible following intravenous gadolinium administration.[3,13] The initial contrast-enhanced images should be obtained in the axial plane, parallel to the operated disc space levels, and with fat-suppression technique in the absence of surgical hardware at the operated levels. Finally, it is important to be aware that significant epidural fibrosis and scarring, without a true disc herniation, may result in recurrent or persistent radiculitis, and therefore, require clinical management including possible reoperation.[1,3,9,13,14]

Frank reherniations may, of course, be identified after surgery. When a recurrent or residual disc herniation is present, it is not necessarily responsible for the patient's symptoms. One study of asymptomatic patients showed residual or recurrent disc herniation in 24% of patients at the operated level within 6 weeks of surgery. In 16% of these asymptomatic patients there was mild to moderate mass effect on the dural sac, whereas 5% had severe compression of the dural sac. Equally important to remember is that herniated disc fragments can regress spontaneously over time.[1,9,13]

Evaluation After Instrumentation

Initial evaluation of the spine following placement of orthopedic hardware should include a detailed description of the type of hardware used and its exact location within the spine. This exact location is imperative to the spine surgeon in evaluating whether the instrumentation was placed in the appropriate spinal levels as planned before the surgical procedure. Prior imaging studies, if available, should be evaluated to assess whether the initial problem at hand has been addressed. Equally important is to assess whether there are hardware-related complications such as implant malpositioning, implant loosening, and implant fracture.[1,3,9,14,15] The spinal alignment should also be carefully scrutinized. Postsurgical malalignment may reflect unexpected changes in weight-bearing distribution or implant malpositioning resulting in spinal instability. In the early postoperative period such a condition may require surgical revision and therefore should be reported to the surgeon.

When evaluating posterior spinal hardware special attention should be given to pedicle screws, which are often used as anchoring devices in spinal fusion and stabilization procedures. Optimal pedicle screw placement is when the screw traverses the central portion of the pedicle and is parallel to the vertebral endplate (Fig. 6).[1,3] Complications include medial angulation of the screw, which may lead to disruption of the medial cortex of the pedicle and nerve root irritation. Lateral angulation may also occur and is especially important in the cervical spine, where the screw may traverse the foramen transversarium and potentially compromise the vertebral artery. Improper placement may also lead to screws traversing the anterior cortex of the vertebral body, sometimes abutting the aorta. Similarly, when evaluating anterior plate and screw fixation the screws may overpenetrate and lead to dural, cord, or nerve root injury (Fig. 7). Such complications can be avoided by using intraoperative fluoroscopy and pedicle screw electrical stimulation to confirm appropriate screw positioning.[1–3,14,15]

Implant loosening is often due to osseous resorption around the anchoring screws. Loosening, as can be identified by increased lucency adjacent to the surgical implants, allows increased motion, which results in a positive feedback cycle of progressive resorption and increased motion (Fig. 8). This cycle eventually leads to destruction of the adjacent osseous structures and complete failure of the implant because of fractures or screw pullout. Hardware fracture or dislodgment is often associated with regional motion and spinal

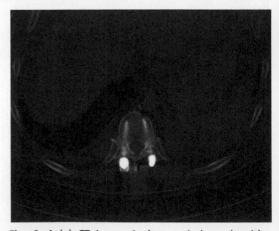

Fig. 6. Axial CT image in bone window algorithm demonstrating optimal pedicle screw positioning. The screw traverses the body of the pedicle without lateral or medial angulation. The vertebral cortex is not disrupted. The screw is parallel to the vertebral body endplate in the sagittal plane (not shown).

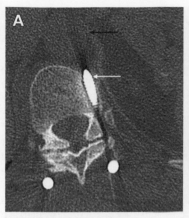
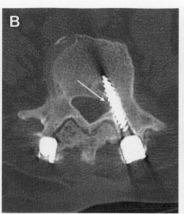
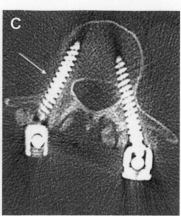

Fig. 7. Suboptimal pedicle screw positioning. Axial CT images in bone window algorithm demonstrating the left pedicle screw breeching the vertebral cortex (*white arrow*) anteriorly (*A*). Notice the close proximity of the screw tip to the aorta (*black arrow*). Axial CT image (*B*) demonstrating a left pedicle screw breeching medial aspect of pedicle cortex and encroaching on the lateral recess. Axial CT image (*C*) demonstrating a right pedicle screw breeching the right lateral cortex of the pedicle and vertebral body (*white arrow*).

instability, which may be the result of or cause of pseudoarthrosis. Implant failure is crucial to detect because timely diagnosis may prevent exacerbation of the underlying pathologic conditon and allow for surgical repair. In certain cases, fractured hardware may not be displaced, making detection of such a complication more difficult.[3,14,15]

A key component of interbody spinal fusion is the interbody spacer. It is important to monitor spacer position in both the horizontal and the vertical planes on serial imaging studies (**Fig. 9**). For this purpose, lucent spacers are fitted with radiopaque markers delineating the spacer's position.

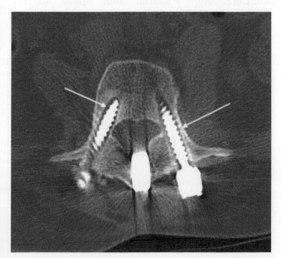

Fig. 8. A 47-year-old female patient after lumbar spinal fusion with low back pain. Axial CT image in bone window algorithm demonstrates increased lucency (*white arrows*) adjacent to bilateral pedicle screws within the L4 vertebral body, consistent with loosening.

A posterior marker located approximately 2 mm anterior to the posterior edge of the adjacent vertebral body indicates the spacer is in a good position and that there is no retropulsion.[1,2] Regarding the vertical plane, a certain degree of cage subsidence is expected and may allow for better fusion. However, excessive subsidence results in a loss of the intervertebral disc space and narrowing of the neural foramen, which may in turn lead to radicular symptoms.[3] This finding should be discussed with the spine surgeon.

It is important to evaluate the soft tissues adjacent to implanted hardware. In the cervical spine, an anterior approach is associated with increased risk of injury to the esophagus, trachea, lungs, and the carotid arteries. Similarly, using an anterior approach in the thoracic or lumbar spine can place the aorta, inferior vena cava, and other abdominal and pelvic structures at an increased risk for injury. Surgical hardware may also dislodge and impinge on adjacent soft tissue structures. Posteriorly, this may lead to chronic soft tissue ulceration and subsequent infections.[3]

Adjacent segment disease
Following spinal fusion, the spinal segments cranial or caudal to the surgical bed are at increased risk for accelerated degeneration due to a shift in the weight-bearing load away from the fused segments to the adjacent vertebrae and reduction in overall flexibility and motion of the spine.[1,3] The persistent increased stress at the perisurgical levels often manifests in premature degenerative changes and may progress to single or multilevel spinal stenosis requiring further operative management. Adjacent segment disease is more

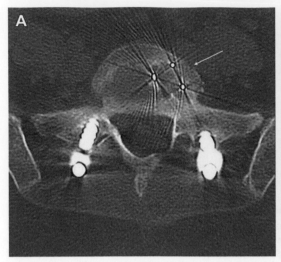
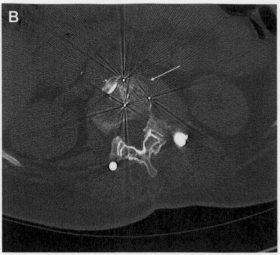

Fig. 9. Malpositioned interbody spacers. Two axial CT images (*A, B*) in bone window algorithm from different patients demonstrating left lateral displacement of an interbody spacer (*white arrows*). Comparison is made with Fig. 3, where the spacer is located centrally relative to the vertebral column.

common in the lumbar spine and most often observed in the cranial perisurgical level, as the superior spine is leveraged against the fused segment.[3] Regardless of the location, early detection of adjacent segment disease is important.

Foreign body

Misplaced foreign bodies may be detected on imaging of patients after spinal surgery. Although detection of misplaced metal hardware or surgical instruments is usually quite simple, a misplaced sponge may elude detection even by an experienced radiologist and especially on MR imaging. Modern surgical sponges do indeed contain a radiopaque filament (composed of barium sulfate), which allows for detection on CT and plain films. However, this filament is neither magnetic nor paramagnetic and therefore cannot be detected on MR imaging.[1] Intraoperative sponge counts by the surgical team are therefore critical with respect to alerting the radiologist about a possible retained foreign body.

On MR imaging, a lesion composed of cotton-like material demonstrates low signal intensity on both T1- and T2-weighted images (a small area of central high signal may, however, be observed on T2 if central necrosis occurs). Contrast administration yields a peripherally enhancing mass, presumably related to a peripheral inflammatory foreign body reaction.[1] Such a lesion may be confused with a postoperative fibrotic reaction, postoperative abscess formation, or the development of a local mass. Correlation with additional imaging as well the clinical presentation of the

patient is therefore crucial in making the correct diagnosis.

GENERAL COMPLICATIONS

At times spinal surgery may result in what is termed failed back surgery syndrome. This syndrome is characterized by residual pain and functional disability after spinal surgery and is often thought to be a result of residual disc herniation, arachnoiditis, radiculitis, or a failure to identify the initial underlying structural problem preoperatively.[1] Patients after spinal surgery, however, may present with a host of additional

Table 1	
Spine surgery complications	
Early	
Postoperative fluid collection	Hematoma, seroma, pseudomeningocele
Operative injury	Fracture, neural injury, vascular injury
Late	
Inflammation	Arachnoiditis, radiculitis
Infection	Spondylodiscitis
Acceleration of degenerative disease	Adjacent level disease
Instrumentation failure	Fractured screw or rod
Fusion failure	Pseudoarthrosis

complications that are crucial to patient management and must be identified on imaging studies. These complications may be stratified to early and late complications as detected on imaging (Table 1). The presence of a potential complication should immediately be discussed with the spine surgeon at the time of the study, with appropriate documentation in the radiology report.[1,3,13,14,16]

SUMMARY

Evaluation of the postoperative spine is a complex task that requires a detailed approach by the radiologist. First, the interpreting radiologist must appreciate the clinical presentation of the patient. Second, it is crucial to be familiar with the instrumentation and operative techniques used by the surgeon. Third, one must be familiar with both the expected postoperative changes and the complications that may be encountered following spinal surgery. It is only through a comprehensive clinical, surgical, and radiologic understanding that a proper evaluation of the postoperative spine can be rendered.

REFERENCES

1. Von Goethem JW, Parizel PM, Jinkins JR. Review article: MRI of the postoperative lumbar spine. Neuroradiology 2002;44:723–39.
2. Rutherford EE, Tarplett LJ, Davies EM, et al. Lumbar spine fusion and stabilization: hardware, techniques, and imaging appearances. Radiographics 2007;27(6):1737–49.
3. Thakkar RS, Malloy JP 4th, Thakkar SC, et al. Imaging the postoperative spine. Radiol Clin North Am 2012;50(4):731–47.
4. Eliyas JK, Karahalios D. Surgery for degenerative lumbar spine disease. Dis Mon 2011;57(10):592–606.
5. Slone RM, MacMillan M, Montgomery WJ. Spinal fixation. Part 1. Principles, basic hardware, and fixation techniques for the cervical spine. Radiographics 1993;13(2):341–56.
6. Slone RM, MacMillan M, Montgomery WJ, et al. Spinal fixation. Part 2. Fixation techniques and hardware for the thoracic and lumbosacral spine. Radiographics 1993;13(3):521–43.
7. Slone RM, McEnery KW, Bridwell KH, et al. Fixation techniques and instrumentation used in the thoracic, lumbar, and lumbosacral spine. Radiol Clin North Am 1995;33(2):233–65.
8. Murtagh RD, Quencer RM, Castellvi AE, et al. New techniques in lumbar spinal instrumentation: what the radiologist needs to know. Radiology 2011; 260(2):317–30.
9. Herrera Herrera I, Moreno de la Presa R, González Gutiérrez R, et al. Evaluation of the postoperative lumbar spine. Radiology 2013;55(1):12–23.
10. Ross JS, Zepp R, Modic MT. The postoperative lumbar spine: enhanced MR evaluation of the intervertebral disk. AJNR Am J Neuroradiol 1996;17(2): 323–31.
11. Hegde V, Meredith DS, Kepler CK. Management of postoperative spinal infections. World J Orthop 2012;3(11):182–9.
12. Leone A, Cerase A, Lauro L, et al. Postoperative lumbar spine. Rays 2000;25(1):125–36.
13. Dina TS, Boden SD, Davis DO. Lumbar spine after surgery for herniated disk: imaging findings in the early postoperative period. AJR Am J Roentgenol 1995;164(3):665–71.
14. Hancock CR, Quencer MR, Falcone S. Challenges and pitfalls in postoperative spine imaging. Appl Radiol 2008;37:23–34.
15. Hayashi D, Roemer FW, Mian A, et al. Imaging features of postoperative complications after spinal surgery and instrumentation. AJR Am J Roentgenol 2012;199(1):W123–9.
16. Douglas-Akinwande AC, Buckwalter KA, Rydberg J, et al. Multichannel CT: evaluating the spine in postoperative patients with orthopedic hardware. Radiographics 2006;26:97–110.

Postoperative Spine Complications

Morgan C. Willson, MD[a],*, Jeffrey S. Ross, MD[b]

KEYWORDS

- Imaging • Postoperative spine • Complications • Surgery

KEY POINTS

- Imaging of the postoperative spine and associated complications is a common clinical scenario for the radiologist; however, despite advanced imaging techniques and better spatial resolution, this remains a challenging task.
- Evaluation of the postoperative spine requires a general knowledge of the surgical approach to each spinal region and the normal temporal evolution of expected postoperative changes.
- Knowledge of specific complications relating to each surgical approach and an understanding of general complications common among various surgical procedures, such as the appropriate evaluation of postoperative hardware, will assist the radiologist in interpretation of postoperative fusion and complications.

INTRODUCTION

Back pain is one of the most common clinical complaints in medicine. Low back pain affects up to 80% of the population during their lifetime and 1% to 2% of the United States population is disabled by low back pain.[1,2] In 2002 the National Health Interview Study sampled 36,161 households, and found that back pain within the last 3 months was the most frequent type of pain reported with 26.4% of the respondents.[3] The rate of spine surgery in the United States is the highest in the world, more than 1.2 million spinal surgeries being performed each year, although there is high geographic variation suggesting poor professional consensus on treatment approaches. For example, Medicare data for 2001 show a 6-fold variation in spine surgery rates among United States cities and a 10-fold variation in the rate of spinal fusion.[4–6]

Postoperative complications may be immediately apparent after surgery or delayed by weeks, months, or years. The overall incidence of major neurologic deficit immediately after spinal surgery is low, with an overall incidence of less than 1%, and slightly more common after thoracic spine surgery (0.49%), followed by the cervical (0.29%) and lumbar spine, respectively (0.08%).[7] The etiology of major neurologic injury during spinal surgery can include direct surgical trauma to the cord or neural elements, compression and/or distraction of the vertebral column, vascular compromise (local infarct or systemic hypotension), epidural and subdural hematoma, and mechanical compression from infolding of the ligamentum flavum, posterior longitudinal ligament, disc, or adjacent bony structures. Over time an estimated 10% to 20% of patients will experience 1 or more complications relating to surgery, and imaging plays an important role in preoperative assessment and postoperative management.

Routine scheduled postoperative imaging may be performed in otherwise asymptomatic patients to evaluate the position and appearance of spinal

Funding Sources: None.
Conflict of Interest: None.
[a] Department of Radiology, Foothills Medical Center, 1403 29th Street Northwest, Calgary, Alberta T2N 2T9, Canada; [b] Neuroradiology Department, Barrow Neurologic Institute, St Joseph's Hospital and Medical Center, 350 West Thomas Road, Phoenix, AZ 85013, USA
* Corresponding author.
E-mail address: mwillson77@gmail.com

Neuroimag Clin N Am 24 (2014) 305–326
http://dx.doi.org/10.1016/j.nic.2014.01.002

instrumentation or to assess the progression of spinal fusion. Alternatively, imaging is often performed to assess immediate or delayed postoperative complications in the symptomatic patient and to further evaluate patients with little or no relief of symptoms following the initial surgical procedure; the so-called failed back surgery syndrome.

SURGICAL APPROACHES AND SPECIFIC RELATED COMPLICATIONS

Multiple surgical techniques are available to access the spinal osseous elements, spinal cord, nerve roots, and intervertebral disc. The individual techniques may vary by region and underlying abnormality. However, the basic goal of each technique is similar: to facilitate safe access to the pathologic area of interest and minimize potential risk. In general, spinal surgeries can be categorized as decompressive or spinal stabilization/fusion procedures, although many examples are a combination of both. Decompressive procedures include discectomy, laminotomy, laminectomy, and facetectomy to decompress a stenotic spinal canal or neural foramen. Spinal fusion allows stabilization of spinal segments for developmental, degenerative, and posttraumatic instability, or iatrogenic causes of instability such as prior surgery.

Cervical Spine Approaches

Anterior cervical approach

The transoral-transpharyngeal approach allows access to the anterior clivus, C1, and C2 for a variety of abnormalities including basilar invagination, odontoid fractures or nonunion, rheumatoid arthritis with cranial settling and/or pannus formation, developmental disorders such as os odontoidium and odontoid hypoplasia, and tumors.[8] The alternative approach to the anterior spine is via a retropharyngeal technique. The anteromedial approach uses the space between the carotid sheath laterally and the sternocleidomastoid muscle and tracheoesophageal complex medially, whereas an anterolateral approach goes lateral to the carotid sheath.

Although rare, occurring in less than 0.2% of anterior cervical discectomy and fusion (ACDF) surgeries, one of the most feared complications related to the anterior cervical approach is direct spinal cord injury. Spinal cord impingement or direct spinal cord trauma may result from vertebral body screws that extend too far through the posterior cortex. However, the risk of spinal cord injury is higher when instruments are advanced into the spinal canal from the anterior approach to remove

posterior osteophytes.[9,10] Plain radiographs and/or computed tomography (CT) will show misplacement of screws or other hardware that impinge or traverse the spinal cord. On magnetic resonance (MR) imaging spinal cord contusion or laceration is manifest, with focal areas of T2 hyperintensity within the spinal cord. If there is associated hemorrhage, gradient recalled echo sequences may show foci of susceptibility within the spinal cord.

The most common reported complications associated with anterior cervical approaches include postoperative dysphagia, postoperative hematoma, and recurrent laryngeal nerve palsy. Dural leak and esophageal perforation are additional less common, but clinically important complications related to the anterior cervical approach.[9] Although postoperative dysphagia is common, imaging of the neck is often normal unless there is clear evidence of hardware failure or malpositioning that results in impingement on the esophagus and adjacent soft tissues (Fig. 1). A barium esophagram may show luminal narrowing during dynamic visualization of swallowing or delayed transit.[11]

Injury to the vertebral artery, estimated to occur in 0.25% of anterior cervical discectomies, may occur following removal of bone too far laterally or lateral placement of hardware.[12-14] The location of cervical hardware is best evaluated on CT. If vertebral artery injury is suspected intraoperatively or the patient presents with new neurologic deficits, initial evaluation with CT angiography will allow direct evaluation of hardware positioning and evaluation for potential vascular injury. There may be localized irregularity with or without narrowing, or demonstration of a dissection flap. Long tapered narrowing or occlusion is highly suggestive of dissection. Alternatively, vascular imaging may show focal pseudoaneurysm or active contrast extravasation.

Posterior cervical approach

A posterior approach to the cervical spine allows direct access to the posterior elements and the potential for wide exposure. A laminotomy, laminectomy, or laminoplasty can be performed to treat multilevel degenerative spondylosis, soft disc herniation, and ossification of the posterior longitudinal ligament.

The major complications associated with the posterior cervical approach include new transient or permanent cervical radiculopathy, vertebral artery injury, and progressive postlaminectomy kyphosis.

The placement of posterior fusion hardware in the cervical spine differs from that in the thoracic and lumbar spine. The pedicles in the cervical

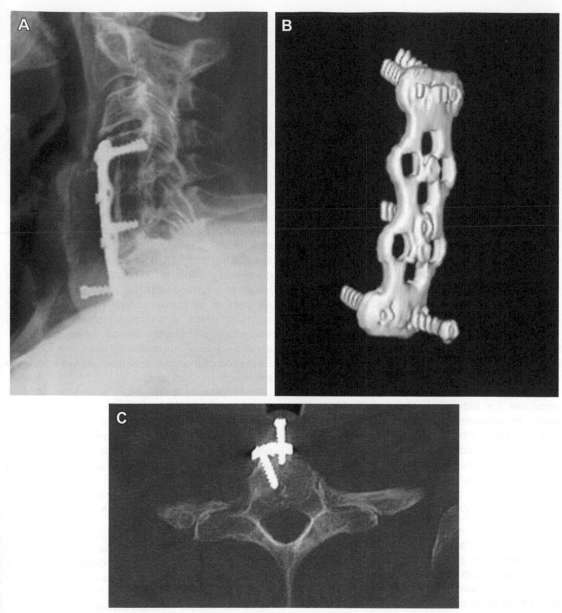

Fig. 1. Anterior cervical discectomy and fusion from C4 to C7. (*A*) Lateral radiograph. Three-dimensional reformatted computed tomography (CT) image (*B*) and axial CT image with bone window algorithm (*C*) show that the C7 screw on the left has backed out from its expected position flush with the cervical plate.

spine are small from C3 to C6 and larger at C2 and C7. Therefore, posterior cervical fusion typically involves lateral mass screws from C3 to C6, with traditional pedicle screws being reserved for the larger C2 and C7 levels. Direct impingement by osseous fragments or malposition of spinal hardware may result in new cervical radiculopathy, best visualized on CT. Other causes of new postoperative radiculopathy, including distraction of neural elements, direct trauma during surgery, and symptomatic hematoma, may require MR imaging for visualization. The rate of vertebral artery injury with the posterior cervical approach is less than 1% and is usually secondary to malposition of lateral mass or pedicle screws.

The rate of postoperative kyphosis varies widely, although it is clearly higher in patients who do not undergo fusion and those with spinal cord dysfunction. Kyphosis is easily evaluated with radiographs, and flexion-extension views may also be helpful to determine the degree of physiologic dysfunction.

Thoracic Approaches

Thoracic disc herniations represent less than 1% of symptomatic spinal disc herniations, although there is a high incidence of incidental disc herniations visualized on MR imaging (>15%). Unlike cervical and lumbar laminectomy, there is a relatively high incidence of neurologic injury with a posterior laminectomy in the thoracic spine and, therefore, procedures are designed to approach the pathologic region as directly as possible with minimal manipulation of the spinal cord. In general, approaches to the thoracic spine are considered anterior and posterolateral. Anterior approaches include a variety of transthoracic procedures as well as the thoracoscopic approach. Posterior and posterolateral approaches include transpedicular (with or without endoscopy), transfacet, and transforaminal, in addition to costotransversectomy and lateral extracavitary approaches.

Intraoperative localization of thoracic vertebral levels remains a specific concern in thoracic spine surgery. Indeed, a 2008 questionnaire study found that nearly 50% of spine surgeons surveyed reported a wrong level surgery during their career.[15] A variety of factors including overlying scapular shadows, variation in the number of rib-bearing vertebrae, and osteopenia all contribute to the difficulty in accurately localizing specific thoracic vertebral levels intraoperatively. To avoid this potential complication, preoperative placement of radiopaque markers using fluoroscopy or CT at the pedicle of interest may be helpful.[16,17]

Lumbar Approaches

Anterior lumbar approaches

Anterior lumbar interbody fusion (ALIF) is typically performed when posterior decompression is not required and pain is the predominant symptom. With a lower abdominal or retroperitoneal approach through the flank, disc material is removed and disc height restored with interbody spacers. Stabilization is most commonly supplemented with an anterior metallic plate and vertebral screws, although occasionally lateral or posterior instrumentation is used. Complications specific to the anterior lumbar approach include vascular injury and retrograde ejaculation. The incidence of vascular complications shows a variable range in the literature, although a recent review suggests an incidence of less than 5%.[18] Overall, vascular injury is more common during laparoscopic procedures than during open ALIF, and venous laceration is more common than arterial injury. Visceral injury such as bowel perforation is rare.[19] Retrograde ejaculation is associated with manipulation of the autonomic plexus, which is closely associated with the aorta

and vena cava at the bifurcation, and drapes over the ventral surface of the spine and sacral body. Rates of retrograde ejaculation vary up to 7.2% in the literature, with higher rates noted in cases using human recombinant bone morphogenic protein 2.[20–22]

Posterior lumbar approaches

Posterior lumbar discectomy without fusion is used to decompress the disc space for treatment of disc herniation. The standard open discectomy involves laminotomy or hemilaminectomy, resection of the ligamentum flavum, and retraction of neural elements, allowing access to the disc space and excision of disc material.

Posterior lumbar interbody fusion (PLIF) involves wide bilateral laminectomies and partial facetectomy. With distraction of the vertebral segment, discectomy is performed and restoration of disc height is achieved with bone graft (autologous or allograft) or synthetic materials such as polymer cages or metal. A common variation of PLIF is transforaminal lumbar interbody fusion (TLIF) with a posterolateral approach through the foramen. Resection of the ipsilateral facet allows access to the thecal sac and disc.

Posterolateral fusion (PLF) is an alternative or supplement to PLIF whereby bone graft is placed laterally between the transverse processes rather than between the vertebral bodies. PLF is used primarily when there is severe loss of disc height, and insertion of an interbody spacer may result in neurologic compromise. PLF is usually supplemented by posterior instrumentation such as pedicle screws and stabilization rods.

Lateral and axial interbody fusion

Extreme lateral interbody fusion and axial interbody fusion have also been described. This far lateral approach places the lumbosacral plexus at risk of injury, as well as the genitofemoral nerve that lies in the psoas muscle. The most common complication associated with this approach is anterior thigh pain and weakness of hip flexors.[23–26]

COMPLICATIONS OF HARDWARE DEVICES AND INSTRUMENTATION

A familiarity with the commonly used devices and instrumentation used in the spine is important for the evaluation of the adequacy of hardware positioning and the assessment of complications such as hardware failure, device migration, or loosening.

It is important to stress that the instrumentation used in spinal fusion is used as an adjunct to bony fusion, to decrease the incidence of pseudarthrosis and to stabilize the spine until osseous fusion is complete. Without bony fusion, all devices will eventually fail under physiologic mechanical stress.

Hardware failure results when an implant breaks or is displaced relative to the underlying bone. Fracture of hardware components without significant displacement is best visualized on CT or plain radiographs, as MR imaging is limited because of hardware artifact. Before device failure there is often a preceding phase of loosening related to instability from ongoing motion, pseudarthrosis, or infection. Loosening appears as a rim of lucency surrounding screws or other devices, particularly when this lucency exceeds 2 mm or increases on sequential examinations (Fig. 2).[27,28]

Anterior fixation devices typically consist of an anterior plate anchored to the vertebral body with screws. The plate should be flush with the anterior vertebral body. Screws pass through the anterior cortex and are seated in the posterior cortex without cortical breakthrough. Ideally screws should not enter an adjacent endplate. Screws that extend too far through the posterior cortex may impinge or damage the spinal cord. Other

complications include screws fracturing under stress or backing out of the plate, although many newer constructs include a locking plate with special cannulated screws, and screw caps that lock the plate and screws together preventing the screws from backing out.

As with hardware in other anatomic areas, there can be irritation or impingement on the adjacent soft tissues. In the cervical spine this may cause prevertebral or retropharyngeal inflammation or injury of vascular structures, esophagus, or trachea.

Pedicle screws in the thoracolumbar spine and lateral mass screws in the subaxial cervical spine are commonly used in combination with plates, hooks, or rods for spinal fusion. This approach results in a strong fusion construct and high rates of spinal fusion. The location of pedicle screws and their close proximity to adjacent neural and vascular structures results in a reported complication rate of 2.4% per screw.[29] Optimal screw placement is along the medial aspect of the pedicle without breaching the cortex, entering the neural foramen or extending beyond the vertebral body cortex (Fig. 3).[30] The most common

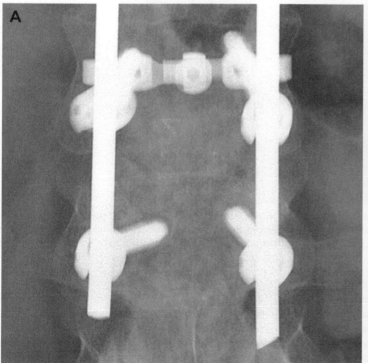
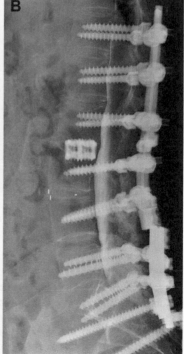

Fig. 2. (A) Frontal radiograph following posterior fusion with bilateral pedicle screws and vertical stabilization rods. There is a thin lucent rim surrounding the lower pedicle screws, which had progressed from prior examinations (not shown), suggesting hardware loosening. (B) Lateral radiograph obtained for lumbar myelogram shows overt fracture of the vertical connecting rods bilaterally in a patient with long-segment posterior fusion of the spine from T12 to S1 and the ilium. In addition, interbody graft prostheses are noted at L2-L3 and L3-L4.

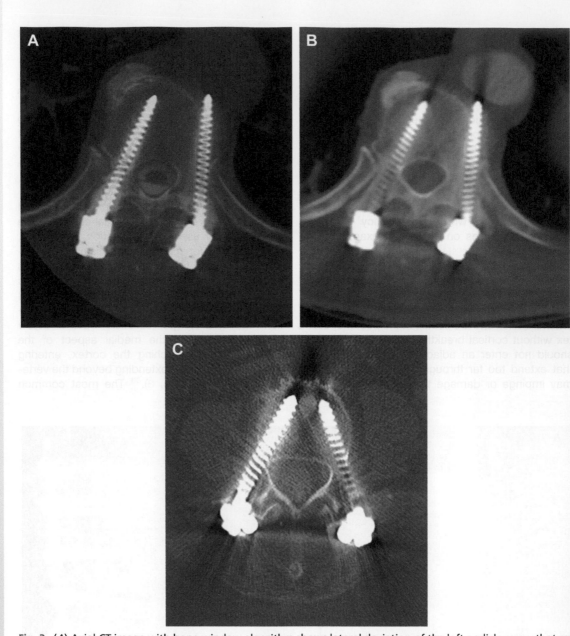

Fig. 3. (A) Axial CT image with bone window algorithm shows lateral deviation of the left pedicle screw that extends beyond the anterolateral cortex. (B) Contrast-enhanced axial CT image in bone window algorithm shows the left pedicle screw contacting the posterior wall of the aorta. (C) Axial CT image shows optimal placement of pedicle screw.

reported complication of pedicle screws is medial angulation of the screw with violation of the medial cortex, resulting in irritation of nerve root.[31]

Interbody fusion may be performed with morselized autografts placed within and/or around bone graft or interbody fusion cages. Although many interbody fusion devices are radiolucent, they can be visualized on radiographs and CT with small radiopaque markers that are contained within the device. The posterior marker should be at least

2 mm anterior to the posterior vertebral body margin to exclude ramp/cage protrusion into the spinal canal.[32]

Total disc replacement (TDR) is performed for discogenic pain without significant spinal stenosis or spondylolisthesis, and has become an increasingly popular alternative to spinal fusion. TDR is used to restore normal mobility and decrease the incidence of accelerated degenerative changes to adjacent segments. As with other new devices, there is a relative paucity of information regarding the complications associated with total disc replacement surgery. A recent review describes an overall complication rate related to the surgical approach (eg, vascular or nerve root injury, retrograde ejaculation) of approximately 2.1% to 18.7% and complications related to the prosthesis (such as migration or displacement, subsidence, implant failure, and endplate fractures) ranging from 2.0% to 39.3%.[33]

As an alternative to traditional decompression, interspinous spacer devices have recently been introduced. These spacers are inserted between the spinous process through a small incision along the interspinous ligament, and function to reduce spinal stenosis by restoring height posteriorly, reducing infolding of the ligamentum flavum and overriding facets.[34] The appearance of specific devices varies slightly, and there may be a hollow component within the spacer for placement of bone graft material, as well as fusion spikes along the wings of the device for attachment to the adjacent spinous process above and below. Complications include posterior migration or extrusion of the device, erosion into the adjacent spinous process, or spinous process fracture that may occur with distraction of the vertebral segment during insertion or during the postoperative course.

PSEUDARTHROSIS

Failure of progression to solid osseous fusion is often the result of ongoing motion. The rate of pseudarthrosis has been reported to be as high as 20% in some series, and risk factors include revision surgery for prior nonunion, chronic illness, smoking, and long-term use of nonsteroidal anti-inflammatory drugs (NSAIDs).[35] In particular, smoking has been shown experimentally to inhibit revascularization and suppress bone formation, and multiple studies have shown increased rates of nonunion in fusion of the cervical and lumbar spine, although the effect is diminished with the use of rigid instrumentation.[35–37] The presence of pseudarthrosis itself may be symptomatic with ongoing microscopic or macroscopic motion, further contributing to degenerative changes. Increased stress on mechanical hardware can ultimately result in failure. Osseous fusion is best demonstrated on serial radiographic assessment or CT, and evaluation is based on the assessment of multiple factors (Box 1).

POSTOPERATIVE INFECTION

The incidence of infection following spinal surgery is low. However, with the increasing number of

---

Box 1
Assessment of radiographic fusion

- Visible bone formation bridging the level of fusion
- No clear lucency traversing the fusion or graft material
- No motion or less than 3° of change in flexion and extension views
- No periprosthetic lucency or halo
- No reactive sclerosis in the graft or adjacent vertebrae
- No fracture of the device, graft, or vertebrae

Data from Venu V, Vertinsky AT, Malfair D, et al. Plain radiograph assessment of spinal hardware. Semin Musculoskelet Radiol 2011;15(2):151–62; and Ray C. Threaded titanium cages for lumbar interbody fusions. Spine 1997;22(6):667–80.

---

total spine surgeries, this is a relatively common indication for imaging of the spine. The use of spinal instrumentation clearly increases the risk for postoperative infections, and infection in the presence of implants is a major diagnostic and therapeutic challenge for surgeons and radiologists.[38] Postoperative infection may occur in the immediate postoperative course or as a late complication, particularly in the setting of spinal instrumentation. Early postoperative bacterial spondylodiscitis likely occurs as a result of direct contamination.[39] Late-onset infections may be secondary to hematogenous seeding, or the sterile inflammatory response around hardware components may stimulate low-virulence organisms to fester.[40]

A recent review of surgical-site infections suggests that the average incidence is approximately 1% after simple discectomy.[41] The risk increases with the presence of spinal instrumentation and predisposing factors such as chronic medical illness (renal failure, diabetes mellitus), intravenous drug use, and immunocompromised states, with an overall incidence between 0.7% and 12%.[38,42–45]

In the postoperative setting, enhancement of lumbar nerve roots may be seen in up to 20% of patients with no recurrent clinical symptoms up to 6 weeks following surgery, but in only 2% of asymptomatic patients at 6 months. Thus the appearance of nerve root enhancement in this setting presumably represents a transient sterile radiculitis.[46] Therefore, nerve root enhancement does not necessarily imply meningitis, and must be interpreted in context with surgical timing and other clinical factors. In addition to nerve root enhancement, imaging signs of meningitis in the spine include vague increased cerebrospinal fluid (CSF) signal intensity, resulting in an indistinct appearance of the spinal cord–CSF interface. There may be clumping of nerve roots and, in severe cases, obliteration of the subarachnoid space with purulent material. Spinal cord signal intensity is often normal; however, T2-weighted/short-tau inversion recovery sequences may show focal and/or diffuse areas of hyperintensity within the spinal cord. Following the intravenous administration of a gadolinium contrast agent, there is leptomeningeal and nerve root enhancement that may be smooth or nodular. There may also be linear or nodular enhancement within the subarachnoid space, related to septations or enhancing inflammatory products and debris.

Normal postoperative changes within the intervertebral disc in asymptomatic patients following discectomy include edematous changes within the vertebral endplates and endplate enhancement. Postoperative enhancement of the endplate is visualized as 2 linear bands paralleling the endplates with or without increased T2 signal intensity within the disc space.[47,48] These changes at the site of discectomy and at the peridural and paraspinal soft tissues can be indistinguishable from infection in the postoperative setting and, therefore, correlation with clinical symptoms and laboratory markers such as white blood cell count, erythrocyte sedimentation rate, and C-reactive protein. In specific instances an image-guided percutaneous aspiration and/or biopsy may be required.

Imaging features that are suggestive of discitis/osteomyelitis include disc space height loss, endplate erosion, and vertebral destruction on radiographs and CT. Imaging of advanced cases shows collapse of the vertebral body. On MR imaging, suspicious features include low T1-weighted signal intensity centered about the intervertebral disc involving the adjacent vertebral bodies with corresponding high T2 signal intensity. There may be diffuse or rim contrast enhancement of the disc space and avid contrast enhancement of the adjacent vertebral marrow. A paraspinal and/or epidural phlegmon or abscess may also be present. This combination of MR imaging findings within the disc space, adjacent vertebral bodies, and paravertebral soft tissues is strongly suggestive of spondylodiscitis (Figs. 4–6).

Postoperative fluid collections within the operative bed may represent seroma in the normal postoperative course, a CSF collection caused by durotomy with CSF leakage, or postoperative abscess with significant overlap in the associated imaging features. All postoperative fluid collections, regardless of cause, may result in compression of the thecal sac or nerve root compression and may be symptomatic.

POSTOPERATIVE HEMATOMA

A common indication for postoperative spine imaging is to rule out hematoma in a patient with new or unresolved symptoms postoperatively. Prospective studies have shown that asymptomatic postoperative spinal epidural hematoma is common, identified in 33% to 100% of patients undergoing lumbar disc or spinal decompression surgery. In addition, spinal epidural hematoma of sufficient magnitude to compress the thecal sac was identified in 58% of patients studied prospectively.[49] However, despite its relatively common occurrence, symptomatic postoperative spinal epidural hematoma, resulting in nerve root compression, spinal canal stenosis, or cauda equina syndrome, is rare, with subsequent surgery for decompression occurring in less than 1%.[50]

Postoperative neurologic recovery from symptomatic spinal epidural hematoma depends on the degree of deficit and early decompression. Postoperative functional recovery with early decompression has been reported in 89% to 95% of patients with incomplete neurologic deficit, compared with 38% to 45% of patients with complete impairment. Therefore, immediate identification and communication of the imaging findings in symptomatic patients with referring clinicians is important.[51,52]

Imaging is best performed using MR, which will better show the size, characteristics, and extent of postoperative hematoma, although a biconvex epidural mass can occasionally be seen on CT, with sagittal reformations that best demonstrate craniocaudal extent (Fig. 7). The MR signal characteristics of intraspinal hematoma vary with the age of blood products. As blood ages, hemoglobin transforms from oxyhemoglobin to deoxyhemoglobin and then methemoglobin, then red blood cells are broken down into ferritin and hemosiderin (Table 1).[53] A hyperacute epidural hematoma that is isointense on T1 and hyperintense on T2 can be difficult to distinguish from CSF, although often there are areas of T2 hypointensity relating to blood-clot retraction and fibrin. As hemoglobin transforms into methemoglobin the associated T1 shortening results in high signal intensity on unenhanced T1 images, although T2 signal intensity can vary depending on the intracellular or extracellular compartment. Peripheral or linear enhancement may also be seen, representing a combination of reactive dural hyperemia, epidural septa, or vessels.

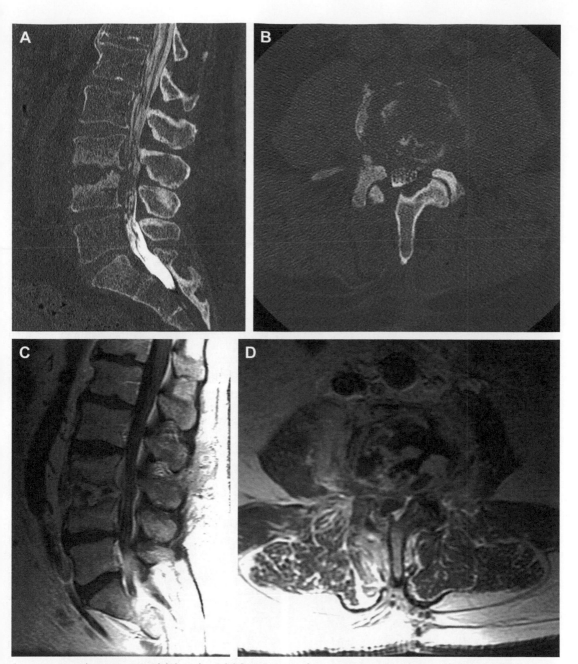

Fig. 4. Postmyelogram sagittal (*A*) and axial (*B*) CT images show postoperative changes following right hemila-minectomy and discectomy at L3-L4 with destruction of the adjacent vertebral endplates and vague associated sclerosis. Sagittal (*C*) and axial (*D*) T1-weighted images after the intravenous administration of gadolinium contrast agent show diffuse enhancement of the L3-L4 intervertebral disc, adjacent vertebral bodies, periverte-bral soft tissues, and bilateral psoas muscles, consistent with discitis-osteomyelitis.

Subdural hematoma is less common than the epidural variety. The appearance is more often clumped or lobulated in appearance, and conforms to the dura. Epidural fat is preserved between the subdural collection and adjacent osseous struc-tures, unlike spinal epidural hematomas.

INFLAMMATORY CHANGES AND SCARRING
Arachnoiditis

Chronic symptoms in 6% to 16% of postsurgical patients have been attributed to arachnoiditis, although the etiology is not well understood.[54]

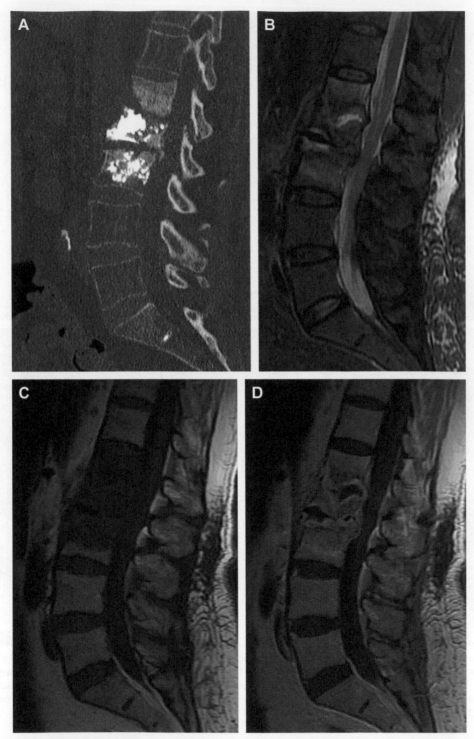

Fig. 5. (*A*) Sagittal CT reformation in bone window algorithm shows vertebral augmentation with acrylic bone cement of the L2 and L3 vertebral bodies. There are superimposed ill-defined destructive changes involving L1-L2. Sagittal short-tau inversion recovery (*B*), sagittal T1-weighted (*C*), and sagittal T1-weighted postgadolinium (*D*) images show diffuse vertebral edema from L1 to L3 with contrast enhancement of the L1-L2 and L2-L3 intervertebral discs and adjacent vertebral bodies. Although better seen on an axial series (not shown), perivertebral soft-tissue contrast enhancement is also noted, and the combination of findings are consistent with discitis-osteomyelitis complicating a prior vertebroplasty procedure.

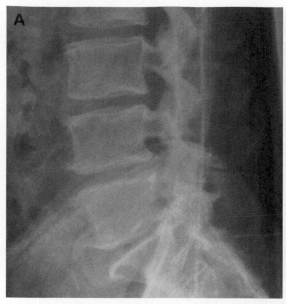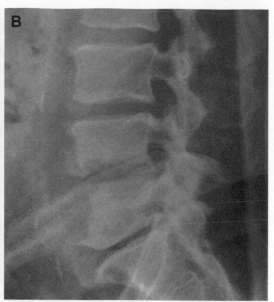

Fig. 6. (*A*) Initial lateral radiograph of the lumbar spine at presentation shows mild multilevel degenerative changes. (*B*) Four weeks following presentation, a repeat lateral radiograph shows irregular destruction of the vertebral endplates at L4-L5, consistent with discitis-osteomyelitis.

Potential factors resulting in arachnoiditis include the surgical procedure itself, intrathecal blood, postoperative infection, prior use of myelographic contrast material or intraspinal injections of anesthetic agents, and use of anti-inflammatory or chemotherapeutic agents.[55]

Three imaging patterns of spinal arachnoiditis have been described, although many cases represent a spectrum with overlapping features.[56] In the first pattern there is central clumping of nerve roots within the thecal sac into a single conglomerate or several thickened cords. The second pattern is the "empty thecal sac" sign. Nerve roots are peripherally displaced and adhered to the meninges, with only the homogeneous T2 hyperintense signal of CSF within the thecal sac (**Fig. 8**). The third pattern of arachnoiditis forms an inflammatory mass that may fill the thecal sac. MR imaging and myelography show a relatively nonspecific soft-tissue mass that may or may not enhance on contrast-enhanced MR imaging studies, depending on the level of active inflammation.

Peridural Fibrosis

In the immediate postoperative period, T1-weighted and T2-weighted MR images show ill-defined soft-tissue infiltration within the epidural space and perineural fat. The postoperative disc is often ill defined secondary to postoperative edema and small amounts of hemorrhage. As a result, in the immediate postoperative period soft tissue and mass effect can be seen in about 80% of patients, often similar in appearance to the preoperative disc herniation.[57] The epidural tissue becomes less prominent over time, and may or may not develop into epidural fibrosis. Peridural fibrosis consists of scar tissue that causes adherence of neural elements to adjacent structures and restricts their mobility. The lack of mobility may cause clinical symptoms or predispose patients to nerve root irritation from the adjacent disc, herniated disc material, or osteophytes. Peridural fibrosis can also cause mass effect and/or direct mechanical compression. Although peridural fibrosis has been implicated in up to 24% of patients with failed back syndrome, the relationship between epidural fibrosis and persistent back or radicular pain is somewhat controversial.[58] Studies have shown that patients with extensive peridural fibrosis are 3.2 times more likely to have recurrent radicular pain,[59] although other studies report no association.[60,61]

CT imaging in the setting of postoperative peridural fibrosis will show nonspecific soft-tissue infiltration with enhancement after intravenous contrast administration. On MR imaging there is infiltrative T1 isointense soft tissue within the epidural space, often along the surgical tract and surrounding nerve roots. Occasionally peridural scar may appear mass-like with effacement of the normal nerve root size or enlargement secondary to cicatrization. After intravenous contrast administration there is diffuse homogeneous enhancement

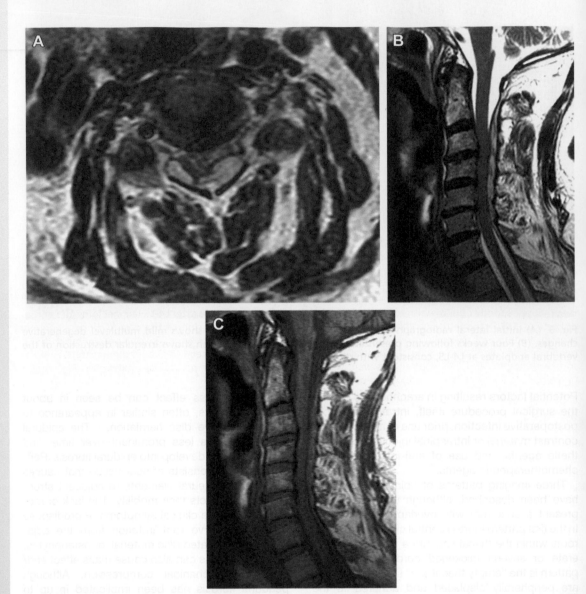

Fig. 7. Axial (*A*) and sagittal (*B*) T2-weighted images show a lobulated posterior epidural fluid collection, mildly hyperintense in comparison with the spinal cord. There is some mass effect on the spinal cord and complete effacement of the surrounding cerebrospinal fluid space. (*C*) Sagittal T1-weighted image shows mild intrinsic T1 hyperintensity, consistent with epidural hematoma with evolving subacute blood products.

Table 1
MR appearance of hematoma

Stage	Age	Hemoglobin	T1, T2 Signal Characteristics
Hyperacute	<12 h	Oxyhemoglobin	Isointense, hyperintense
Acute	1–3 d	Deoxyhemoglobin	Hypointense, hypointense
Early subacute	3–7 d	Intracellular methemoglobin	Hyperintense, hypointense
Late subacute	7–14 d	Extracellular methemoglobin	Hyperintense, hyperintense
Chronic	>2 wk	Hemosiderin	Hypointense, hypointense

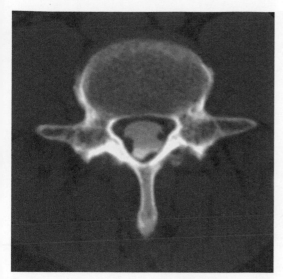

Fig. 8. Axial image of CT performed after the injection of an intrathecal contrast agent shows clumping of the lumbar nerve roots. In addition, the nerve roots are peripherally displaced and adherent to the thecal sac in the setting of arachnoiditis.

that may be present for years after surgery. Occasionally, involved nerve roots may show some degree of enhancement (**Fig. 9**).

With established peridural fibrosis there is no known effective clinical cure. Surgical treatments such as attempted lysis of adhesions are of limited clinical utility. Placement of a spinal cord stimulator may be helpful in select cases. Given the lack of effective treatments, there have been many studies using a variety of materials in attempts to prevent the formation of epidural scar, including autologous fat, synthetic materials such as polytetrafluoroethylene, NSAIDs, and mitomycin.[62–64] Barrier methods including autologous fat, Silastic, Gelfoam, Dacron, and methacrylate, all of which may be visible on imaging studies, have also been used for this purpose, with limited success.

PSEUDOMENINGOCELE, CSF LEAK, AND INTRACRANIAL HYPOTENSION

A CSF leakage syndrome, without or with pseudomeningocele formation, leading to intracranial hypotension is caused by a dural tear or durotomy at the time of surgery. A recent prospective review of cases of elective spine surgery suggests that approximately 3.4% of cases had an incidental durotomy. The incidence was higher in the thoracic (6.6%) and lumbar spine (4.9%) than in the cervical spine (1.3%), and was higher during revision surgery in comparison with primary procedures.[65]

A pseudomeningocele is defined as a CSF-containing cyst in contiguity with the thecal sac, although the dural connection is often difficult to visualize directly on CT or MR imaging. The cyst is not lined by meninges and usually does not contain neural elements, although they may herniate into the cyst occasionally. On CT and MR imaging the density and signal characteristics, respectively, follow that of CSF unless complicated by hemorrhage or infection. There may be a thin rim of peripheral enhancement in uncomplicated cases.

Intracranial findings of CSF leakage syndrome include diffuse dural thickening and enhancement, sagging midbrain, subdural hygroma/hematoma, descent of the cerebellar tonsils, and enlarged veins or dural sinuses (**Fig. 10**). Imaging of the spine may show epidural fluid collections and/or paraspinal fluid, dilation of the epidural venous plexus, and diffuse dural thickening and enhancement.[66–69]

Localization of a CSF leak provides important information for the surgeon to guide further treatment. If there is uncertainty regarding the presence and/or location of a CSF leak, radionuclide cisternography may delineate the site of CSF leak in approximately 55% of cases. Radionuclide cisternography often relies on indirect evidence, such as rapid clearing of radioisotope from the subarachnoid space and early appearance of radiotracer within the bladder. CT myelography may directly visualize the site of leak in approximately 70% of cases or show anatomic abnormalities that predispose to CSF leak. Finally, the investigational use of MR imaging myelography with low-dose intrathecal gadolinium chelate or heavily T2-weighted sequences have also been reported to be helpful, and studies have shown a sensitivity similar to that of CT myelography.[70,71]

Incidental durotomies recognized at the time of surgery are treated with primary closure by sewing the dural edges to form a tight closure. For larger tears or lateral tears, a patch of deep fascia or synthetic material can be used. Treatment of pseudomeningocele and delayed CSF leakage includes CSF diversion by lumbar drainage, fluoroscopic or CT-guided epidural blood patch, primary surgical repair, or oversewing the wound to increase local tissue pressures and tamponade CSF leakage.[72–74]

COMPLICATIONS RELATED TO BONE GRAFT, RECOMBINANT HUMAN BONE MORPHOGENIC PROTEIN, AND HETEROTOPIC BONE

Bone graft material may represent autograft that is harvested from the iliac crest or another source

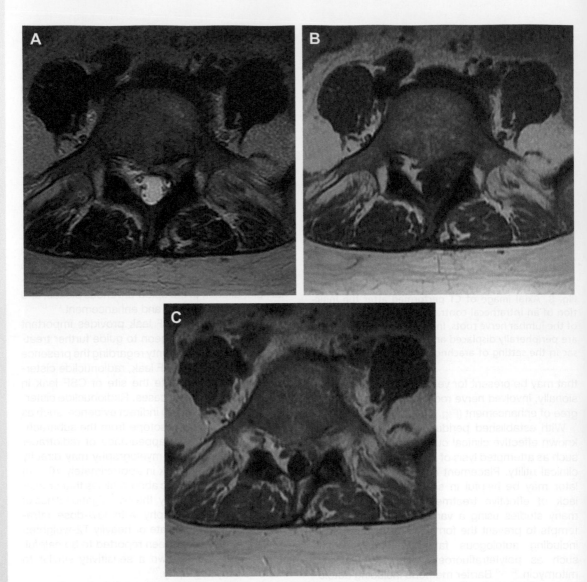

Fig. 9. Axial T2-weighted (*A*) and T1-weighted (*B*) images of a patient with prior left hemilaminectomy for microdiscectomy at L4-L5. There is ill-defined soft tissue of low T2 and T1 signal intensity in the lateral recess surrounding the descending L5 nerve root. (*C*) Diffuse homogeneous enhancement following intravenous gadolinium administration suggesting peridural fibrosis affecting the left L5 nerve root.

such as a rib or bone from the spine removed during surgery, or allograft donor bone that is usually obtained from a tissue bank. Bone graft substitutes including recombinant human bone morphogenic protein (rh-BMP) are also commonly used in the spine. Bone graft can be either structural, used as support for bone or disc that was removed, or onlay (a slurry of bone fragments that grow together to stabilize the spine or bridge a joint). Intraoperative fluoroscopy or radiographs are often used to confirm adequate placement of structural bone grafts. Radiographic follow-up is then performed to assess for progression of fusion and

complications in the postoperative setting. Grafts can migrate over time, become displaced, and even extruded.

BMP is used on label for single-level ALIF with the LT-CAGE device (rhBMP-2 InFUSE; Medtronic Sofamor Danek, Memphis, TN) and with a humanitarian device exemption for use in posterior spine fusions (rhBMP-7 OP-1 Putty; Stryker Biotech, Kalamazoo, MI), although it is often used off label for a variety of spinal fusion procedures.[75,76] BMP enhances arthrodesis following spinal fusion to reduce the 10% to 15% pseudarthrosis rate with iliac crest bone graft and to

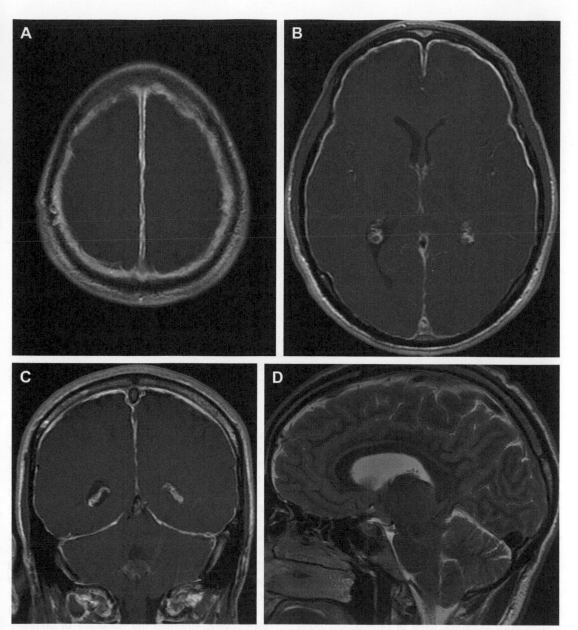

Fig. 10. A 55-year-old woman with persistent positional headache 2 weeks following lumbar puncture. Axial (*A,* *B*) and coronal (*C*) T1-weighted postgadolinium images show diffuse smooth dural thickening and enhancement. In addition, there is mild inferior displacement of the cerebellar tonsils into the foramen magnum. (*D*) Sagittal T2-weighted image shows slumping of the midbrain and pons, downward displacement of brain over the free edge of the incisura, and a distended transverse sinus. These findings, in addition to the clinical history, represent a classic pattern of intracranial hypotension.

reduce the morbidity associated with iliac crest bone graft harvest.[77]

Although osteolysis is a normal part of the re-modeling process leading to fusion, higher rates of resorption have been suggested with BMP that may contribute to migration, displacement, or extrusion of the graft.[78] Radiographic and CT evaluation have been shown to detect endplate resorption in 100% of patients who underwent cervical fusion and 82% of patients after lumbar fusion. In addition, subsidence of the cage resulting in narrowing of the disc space may be seen in more than 50% of cases (**Fig. 11**).[79]

Additional reported complications relating to the use of osteobiologics include extradiscal, ectopic, and heterotopic bone formation, as well as clinical

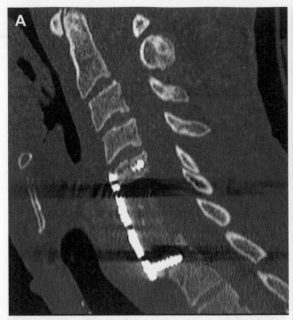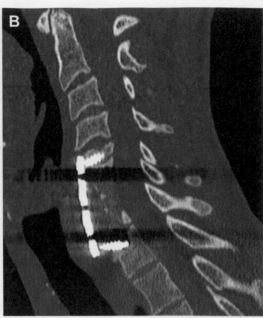

Fig. 11. (A) Sagittal CT reformation in bone window algorithm shows a patient status post anterior cervical fusion with cervical plate extending from C5 to C7 and interposed corpectomy graft. Note that the inferior vertebral body screw extends into the C7-T1 disc and contacts the superior endplate of the T1 vertebral body. (B) On a 2-month follow-up CT scan, there is subsidence of the fusion construct and graft into the superior endplate of the T1 vertebral body.

symptoms associated with new radiculopathy after surgery. Painful seroma, prevertebral edema, and dysphagia are reported with use in the cervical spine, in addition to higher rates of retrograde ejaculation after ALIF.[20,80–84] Heterotopic bone formation often occurs along the TLIF/PLIF tract in the ventrolateral epidural space or the facet complex, resulting in central canal or foraminal stenosis, respectively. On MR imaging the appearance may be variable depending on the presence of dense sclerotic bone or fatty marrow, although the resultant severity of canal or foraminal stenosis is well visualized. CT may be helpful to further characterize potential sites of heterotopic bone suspected on MR imaging, although occasionally extruded graft material can be mistaken for heterotopic bone.

RECURRENT DISC HERNIATION

Recurrent lumbar disc herniation is the most common complication following primary discectomy, and contributes to poor clinical outcomes and increased costs of health care.[85] Recurrent disc herniation is defined by imaging as disc herniation at the level of prior surgery, and may be ipsilateral or contralateral to the previous herniation. Clinically recurrent disc herniation has been defined as recurrent back/leg pain after a definite pain-free interval

lasting at least 6 months from initial surgery. The reported incidence of recurrent disc herniation after lumbar discectomy varies between 3% and 18% in retrospective studies.[86–88] In addition, prospective studies with 2-year serial imaging have found radiographic evidence of recurrent disc herniation in approximately 23% of patients after lumbar discectomy, although almost half of the radiographic disc herniations were asymptomatic.[89]

The accuracy of contrast-enhanced CT and noncontrast MR imaging in the differentiation of recurrent disc herniation and postoperative scar is comparable, approximately 71% and 79%, respectively, whereas the accuracy of contrast-enhanced MR imaging is much higher, approximately 96% to 100%. MR imaging with contrast is therefore the imaging modality of choice in the postoperative lumbar spine (Fig. 12).[90–92]

It is important to differentiate recurrent disc herniation from peridural fibrosis because epidural scar may not benefit from reoperation, whereas the response rate of reoperation for recurrent disc is similar to primary surgical rates.[86] Recurrent disc herniation most often presents as a ventral epidural soft-tissue mass, isointense to parent disc on T1 and isointense to hyperintense to the disc on T2. Disc material shows no enhancement; however, peripheral enhancement is common because of granulation tissue or dilated epidural

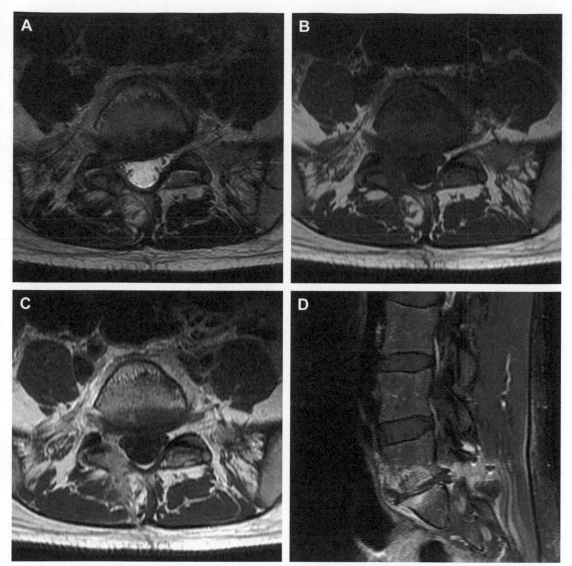

Fig. 12. Axial T2-weighted (*A*) and T1-weighted (*B*) images in a patient with prior right hemilaminectomy for microdiscectomy at L5-S1. There is ill-defined soft tissue of low T2 and T1 signal in the lateral recess surrounding the descending right S1 nerve root. Axial T1-weighted postgadolinium (*C*) and sagittal T1-weighted fat-saturated postgadolinium (*D*) images show peripheral enhancement around the soft tissue in the right lateral recess, consistent with recurrent disc herniation.

plexus. If there is homogeneous diffuse enhancement peridural fibrosis should be favored, although caution is warranted if delayed images are obtained, as contrast may diffuse into disc material from surrounding vascularized scar/granulation tissue and simulate peridural fibrosis.

ACCELERATED JUNCTIONAL/ADJACENT-LEVEL DISEASE

Radiographic adjacent-level disease is often seen following spinal fusion involving either the proximal or distal segment adjacent to fusion. A recent systematic review of the literature suggests that the risk of developing clinically significant adjacent-segment pathology (ASP) after fusion surgery ranges from a cumulative rate of 1.6% to 4.2% per year following cervical fusion and from 0.6% to 3.9% per year after lumbar fusion.[93,94] The risk of ASP in the cervical spine may be higher if there are degenerative changes at C5-C6 or C6-C7 and these levels are adjacent to the surgical level. In the lumbar spine, patients older than 60 years or those with preexisting degenerative disc/facet changes may have an increased risk of ASP. In addition, ASP may be greater after multilevel fusions and fusions adjacent to, but not including, L5-S1.[88,89]

There has been debate in the literature as to whether ASP represents the natural progression of degenerative disease or whether there is accelerated degeneration at levels adjacent to fusion caused by altered mechanics.[95–97] However, biomechanical studies have shown that fusion results in an increase in adjacent-segment range of motion, altered centers of rotation, increased intradiscal pressures, and increased absorption of loads and vibrational stress, and these biomechanical alterations likely play a role in causing adjacent-segment disease.[98] The most common abnormal finding in the adjacent segment is disc degeneration; however, disc herniation, spinal canal stenosis, listhesis, dynamic instability, degenerative facet arthropathy, and foraminal stenosis can all be seen with similar imaging features on MR and CT as degenerative changes in the absence of prior fusion.

REMOTE COMPLICATIONS

Remote complications are those that occur at a distance from, or are unrelated to, the specific operative site. Remote complications include the general risks associated with any surgery such as the risk related to anesthesia, blood loss and/or hypovolemia, myocardial infarction, stroke, pulmonary embolism, deep vein thrombosis, and nosocomial pneumonia. There are, however, 2 remote complications that deserve special attention in relation to spinal surgery.

Intracranial Hemorrhage

Intracranial hemorrhage following spine surgery can occur within the cerebral hemispheres, cerebellum, and subdural or epidural space. The causes of intracranial hemorrhage are uncertain, although most cases involve durotomy or incidental dural tear with loss of CSF, and the most common intracranial compartment involved is the posterior fossa. It is thought that CSF leakage results in sagging of the cerebral hemispheres and cerebellum, which may stretch bridging vascular structures or result in venous compression.[99,100]

Remote cerebellar hemorrhage may present with a varying appearance, although it often appears as striated hyperdense blood (zebra sign) in the cerebellar folia, which may represent a combination of subarachnoid and/or superficial parenchymal hemorrhage. Small hematomas are often treated conservatively, with large hematomas requiring decompression because of mass effect or hydrocephalus.[101]

Ophthalmic Complications

Postoperative ischemic optic neuropathy is a rare but devastating complication that has been described in a variety of surgical procedures, including surgery on the spine.[102] In the setting of postoperative vision loss, urgent ophthalmologic evaluation is recommended to rule out potentially treatable conditions such as acute angle closure glaucoma, retinal detachment, or direct globe injury. In addition, fundoscopic evaluation may assist in the diagnosis of retinal artery occlusion as a cause.[103] The goal of imaging in the setting of postoperative vision loss is to rule out occipital lobe infarct or other causes such as pituitary apoplexy, and ischemic optic neuropathy is often a diagnosis of exclusion. Imaging of the optic nerves is often normal; however, early MR imaging with restricted diffusion along the course of the optic nerve and hyperintense signal on T2-weighted image sequences have been reported.[104]

SUMMARY

Imaging of the postoperative spine and associated complications is a common clinical scenario for the radiologist, although despite advanced imaging techniques and better spatial resolution, this remains a challenging task. Evaluation of the postoperative spine requires a general knowledge of the surgical approach to each spinal region and the normal temporal evolution of expected postoperative changes. Knowledge of specific complications relating to each surgical approach and an understanding of general complications common among various surgical procedures, such as the appropriate evaluation of postoperative hardware, will assist the radiologist in interpretation of postoperative fusion and complications.

REFERENCES

1. Friedly J, Standaert C, Chan L. Epidemiology of spine care: the back pain dilemma. Phys Med Rehabil Clin N Am 2010;21(4):659–77.
2. Deyo RA, Weinstein JN. Low back pain. N Engl J Med 2001;344(5):363–70.
3. Deyo RA, Mirza SK, Martin BI. Back pain prevalence and visit rates. Spine 2006;31(23):2724–7.
4. Weinstein JN, Lurie JD, Olson PR, et al. United States' trends and regional variations in lumbar spine surgery: 1992-2003. Spine 2006;31(23):2707–14.
5. Deyo RA, Mirza SK. Trends and variations in the use of spine surgery. Clin Orthop Relat Res 2006;443(443):139–46.

6. Deyo RA, Mirza SK, Martin BI, et al. Trends, major medical complications, and charges associated with surgery for lumbar spinal stenosis in older adults. JAMA 2010;303(13):1259–65.

7. Cramer DE, Maher PC, Pettigrew DB, et al. Major neurologic deficit immediately after adult spinal surgery. J Spinal Disord Tech 2009;22(8):565–70.

8. Hsu W, Wolinsky JP, Gokaslan ZL, et al. Transoral approaches to the cervical spine. Neurosurgery 2010;66(Suppl 3):119–25.

9. Fountas KN, Kapsalaki EZ, Nikolakakos LG, et al. Anterior cervical discectomy and fusion associated complications. Spine 2007;32(21):2310–7.

10. Kraus D, Stauffer S. Spinal cord injury as a complication of elective anterior cervical fusion. Clin Orthop Relat Res 1975;(112):130–41.

11. Riley LH, Vaccaro AR, Dettori JR, et al. Postoperative dysphagia in anterior cervical spine surgery. Spine 2010;35(Suppl 9):S76–85.

12. Daentzer D, Deinsberger W, Böker DK. Vertebral artery complications in anterior approaches to the cervical spine. Surg Neurol 2003;59(4):299–308.

13. Inamasu J, Guiot BH. Vascular injury and complication in neurosurgical spine surgery. Acta Neurochir 2006;148(4):375–87.

14. Neo M, Sakamoto T, Fujibayashi S, et al. The clinical risk of vertebral artery injury from cervical pedicle screws inserted in degenerative vertebrae. Spine 2005;30(24):2800–5.

15. Mody MG, Nourbakhsh A, Stahl DL, et al. The prevalence of wrong level surgery among spine surgeons. Spine 2008;33(2):194–8.

16. Upadhyaya CD, Wu JC, Chin CT, et al. Avoidance of wrong-level thoracic spine surgery: intraoperative localization with preoperative percutaneous fiducial screw placement. J Neurosurg Spine 2012;16(3):280–4.

17. Binning MJ, Schmidt MH. Percutaneous placement of radiopaque markers at the pedicle of interest for preoperative localization of thoracic spine level. Spine 2010;35(19):1821–5.

18. Wood KB, Devine J, Fischer D, et al. Vascular injury in elective anterior lumbosacral surgery. Spine 2010;35(9):66–75.

19. Rajaraman V, Vingan R, Roth P, et al. Visceral and vascular complications resulting from anterior lumbar interbody fusion. J Neurosurg 1999;91(Suppl 1):60–4.

20. Carragee EJ, Mitsunaga KA, Hurwitz EL, et al. Retrograde ejaculation after anterior lumbar interbody fusion using rhBMP-2: a cohort controlled study. Spine J 2011;11(6):511–6.

21. Lindley EM, McBeth ZL, Henry SE, et al. Retrograde ejaculation after anterior lumbar spine surgery. Spine 2012;37(20):1785–9.

22. Sasso RC, Burkus K, Lehuec J. Retrograde ejaculation after anterior lumbar interbody fusion: transperitoneal versus retroperitoneal. Spine J 2002;2:55S.

23. Cummock MD, Vanni S, Levi AD, et al. An analysis of postoperative thigh symptoms after minimally invasive transpsoas lumbar interbody fusion. J Neurosurg Spine 2011;15(1):11–8.

24. Houten JK, Alexandre LC, Nasser R, et al. Nerve injury during the transpsoas approach for lumbar fusion. J Neurosurg Spine 2011;15(3):280–4.

25. Hu WK, He SS, Zhang SC, et al. An MRI study of psoas major and abdominal large vessels with respect to the X/DLIF approach. Eur Spine J 2011;20(4):557–62.

26. Ahmadian A, Deukmedjian AR, Abel N, et al. Analysis of lumbar plexopathies and nerve injury after lateral retroperitoneal transpsoas approach: diagnostic standardization. J Neurosurg Spine 2013;18(3):289–97.

27. Slone RM, MacMillan M, Montgomery WJ, et al. Spinal fixation part 2: fixation techniques and hardware for the thoracic and lumbosacral spine. Radiographics 1993;13:521–43.

28. Slone RM, MacMillan M, Montgomery WJ. Spinal fixation part 3: complications of spinal instrumentation. Radiographics 1993;13:797–816.

29. Lonstein J, Denis F, Perra J, et al. Complications associated with pedicle screws. J Bone Joint Surg Am 1999;81(11):1519–28.

30. Venu V, Vertinsky AT, Malfair D, et al. Plain radiograph assessment of spinal hardware. Semin Musculoskelet Radiol 2011;15(2):151–62.

31. Young PM, Berquist TH, Bancroft LW, et al. Complications of spinal instrumentation. Radiographics 2007;27(3):775–89.

32. Nouh MR. Spinal fusion-hardware construct: basic concepts and imaging review. World J Radiol 2012;4(5):193–207.

33. Van Den Eerenbeemt KD, Ostelo RW, van Royen BJ, et al. Total disc replacement surgery for symptomatic degenerative lumbar disc disease: a systematic review of the literature. Eur Spine J 2010;19:1262–80.

34. Nandakumar A, Clark N, Smith F, et al. Two-year results of X-Stop interspinous implant for the treatment of lumbar spinal stenosis: a prospective study. J Spinal Disord Tech 2012;26(1):1–7.

35. Suda K, Ito M, Abumi K, et al. Radiological risk factors of pseudarthrosis and/or instrument breakage after PLF with the pedicle screw system in isthmic spondylolisthesis. J Spinal Disord Tech 2006;19(8):541–6.

36. Bose B. Anterior cervical instrumentation enhances fusion rates in multilevel reconstruction in smokers. J Spinal Disord 2001;14(1):3–9.

37. Eubanks JD, Thorpe SW, Cheruvu VK, et al. Does smoking influence fusion rates in posterior cervical

arthrodesis with lateral mass instrumentation? Clin Orthop Relat Res 2011;469(3):696–701.

38. Gerometta A, Rodriguez Olaverri JC, Bitan F. Infections in spinal instrumentation. Int Orthop 2012; 36(2):457–64.

39. Tronnier V, Schneider R, Kunz U, et al. Postoperative spondylodiscitis: results of a prospective study about the aetiology of spondylodiscitis after operation for lumbar disc herniation. Acta Neurochir 1992;117:149–52.

40. Quaile A. Infections associated with spinal implants. Int Orthop 2012;36(2):451–6.

41. Hamdan TA. Postoperative disc space infection after discectomy: a report on thirty-five patients. Int Orthop 2012;36(2):445–50.

42. Pull ter Gunne AF, Hosman AJ, Cohen DB, et al. A methodological systematic review on surgical site infections following spinal surgery: part 1: risk factors. Spine 2012;37(24):2017–33.

43. Van Middendorp JJ, Pull ter Gunne AF, Schuetz M, et al. A methodological systematic review on surgical site infections following spinal surgery: part 2: prophylactic treatments. Spine 2012;37(24):2034–45.

44. Gerometta A, Bittan F, Rodriguez Olaverri JC. Postoperative spondilodiscitis. Int Orthop 2012;36(2): 433–8.

45. Pull ter Gunne AF, Mohamed A, Skolasky RL, et al. The presentation, incidence, etiology, and treatment of surgical site infections after spinal surgery. Spine 2010;35(13):1323–8.

46. Van Goethem JW, Van de Kelft E, Biltjes IG, et al. MRI after successful lumbar discectomy. Neuroradiology 1996;38(Suppl 1):S90–6.

47. Ross JS, Zepp R, Modic MT. The postoperative lumbar spine: enhanced MR evaluation of the intervertebral disk. AJNR Am J Neuroradiol 1996;17(2): 323–31.

48. Bommireddy R, Kamat A, Smith ET, et al. Magnetic resonance image findings in the early postoperative period after anterior cervical discectomy. Eur Spine J 2007;16(1):27–31.

49. Sokolowski M, Garvey T, Perl J, et al. Prospective study of postoperative lumbar epidural hematoma: incidence and risk factors. Spine 2008; 33(1):108–13.

50. Aono H, Ohwada T, Hosono N, et al. Incidence of postoperative symptomatic epidural hematoma in spinal decompression surgery. J Neurosurg Spine 2011;15(2):202–5.

51. Liao CC, Lee ST, Hsu WC, et al. Experience in the surgical management of spontaneous spinal epidural hematoma. J Neurosurg 2004; 100(1 Suppl Spine):38–45.

52. Foo D, Rossier A. Preoperative neurological status in predicting surgical outcome of spinal epidural hematomas. Surg Neurol 1981;15(5):389–401.

53. Braun P, Kazmi K, Nogués-Meléndez P, et al. MRI findings in spinal subdural and epidural hematomas. Eur J Radiol 2007;64(1):119–25.

54. Burton CV, Kirkaldy-Willis WH, Yong-Hing K, et al. Causes of failure of surgery on the lumbar spine. Clin Orthop Relat Res 1981;(157):191–9.

55. Van Goethem JW, Parizel PM, Jinkins JR. Review article: MRI of the postoperative lumbar spine. Neuroradiology 2002;44(9):723–39.

56. Ross J, Masaryk T. MR imaging of lumbar arachnoiditis. AJNR Am J Neuroradiol 1987;149:1025–32.

57. Floris R, Spallone A, Aref T, et al. Early postoperative MRI findings following surgery for herniated lumbar disc part II: a gadolinium-enhanced study. Acta Neurochir 1997;139:1101–7.

58. North R, Campbell J, James C, et al. Failed back surgery syndrome: 5-year follow-up in 102 patients undergoing repeated operation. Neurosurgery 1991;28(5):685–91.

59. Ross J, Robertson J, Fredrickson R, et al. Association between peridural scar and recurrent radicular pain after lumbar discectomy: magnetic resonance evaluation. Neurosurgery 1996;38:855–63.

60. Coskun E, Süzer T, Topuz O, et al. Relationships between epidural fibrosis, pain, disability, and psychological factors after lumbar disc surgery. Eur Spine J 2000;9(3):218–23.

61. Rönnberg K, Lind B, Zoega B, et al. Peridural scar and its relation to clinical outcome: a randomised study on surgically treated lumbar disc herniation patients. Eur Spine J 2008;17(12):1714–20.

62. Sandoval MA, Hernandez-Vaquero D. Preventing peridural fibrosis with nonsteroidal anti-inflammatory drugs. Eur Spine J 2008;17(3):451–5.

63. Ivanic GM, Pink PT, Schneider F, et al. Prevention of epidural scarring after microdiscectomy: a randomized clinical trial comparing gel and expanded polytetrafluoroethylene membrane. Eur Spine J 2006;15(9):1360–6.

64. Çelik SE, Altan T, Çelik S, et al. Mitomycin protection of peridural fibrosis in lumbar disc surgery. J Neurosurg Spine 2008;9(3):243–8.

65. McMahon P, Dididze M, Levi AD. Incidental durotomy after spinal surgery: a prospective study in an academic institution. J Neurosurg Spine 2012; 17(1):30–6.

66. Renowden SA, Gregory R, Hyman N, et al. Spontaneous intracranial hypotension. J Neurol Neurosurg Psychiatr 1995;59:511–5.

67. Dillon W. Spinal manifestations of intracranial hypotension. AJNR Am J Neuroradiol 2001;22:1233–4.

68. Forghani R, Farb RI. Diagnosis and temporal evolution of signs of intracranial hypotension on MRI of the brain. Neuroradiology 2008;50(12): 1025–34.

69. Yousry I, Förderreuther S, Moriggl B, et al. Cervical MR imaging in postural headache: MR signs and

pathophysiological implications. AJNR Am J Neuroradiol 2001;22(7):1239–50.

70. Wang YF, Lirng JF, Fuh JL, et al. Heavily T2-weighted MR myelography vs CT myelography in spontaneous intracranial hypotension. Neurology 2009;73(22):1892–8.

71. Albayram S, Kilic F, Ozer H, et al. Gadolinium-enhanced MR cisternography to evaluate dural leaks in intracranial hypotension syndrome. AJNR Am J Neuroradiol 2008;29(1):116–21.

72. Tosun B, Ilbay K, Kim MS, et al. Management of persistent cerebrospinal fluid leakage following thoraco-lumbar surgery. Asian Spine J 2012;6(3):157–62.

73. Cho KI, Moon HS, Jeon HJ, et al. Spontaneous intracranial hypotension: efficacy of radiologic targeting vs blind blood patch. Neurology 2011;76(13):1139–44.

74. Kranz PG, Gray L, Taylor JN. CT-guided epidural blood patching of directly observed or potential leak sites for the targeted treatment of spontaneous intracranial hypotension. AJNR Am J Neuroradiol 2011;32(5):832–8.

75. U. S. Food and Drug Administration. InFUSE bone graft/LT-CAGE lumbar tapered fusion devices. Approval letter 2002. Available at: http://www.fda.gov/MedicalDevices/ProductsandMedicalProcedures/DeviceApprovalsandClearances/recently-approved devices/ucm083423.htm. Accessed February 10, 2014.

76. U. S. Food and Drug Administration. OP-1 putty. Approval letter 2003. Available at: http://www.fda.gov/medicaldevices/productsandmedicalprocedures/deviceapprovalsandclearances/recently-approved devices/ucm081181.htm. Accessed February 10, 2014.

77. Hsu WK, Wang JC. The use of bone morphogenetic protein in spine fusion. Spine J 2008;8(3):419–25.

78. Helgeson MD, Lehman RA, Patzkowski JC, et al. Adjacent vertebral body osteolysis with bone morphogenetic protein use in transforaminal lumbar interbody fusion. Spine J 2011;11(6):507–10.

79. Sethi A, Craig J, Bartol S, et al. Radiographic and CT evaluation of recombinant human bone morphogenetic protein-2-assisted spinal interbody fusion. AJR Am J Roentgenol 2011;197(1):W128–33.

80. Mroz TE, Wang JC, Hashimoto R, et al. Complications related to osteobiologics use in spine surgery: a systematic review. Spine 2010;35(Suppl 9):S86–104.

81. Benglis D, Wang M, Levi A. A comprehensive review of the safety profile of bone morphogenetic protein in spine surgery. Neurosurgery 2008;62(5 Suppl 2):423–31.

82. Carragee EJ, Hurwitz EL, Weiner BK. A critical review of recombinant human bone morphogenetic protein-2 trials in spinal surgery: emerging safety concerns and lessons learned. Spine J 2011;11(6):471–91.

83. Owens K, Glassman SD, Howard JM, et al. Perioperative complications with rhBMP-2 in transforaminal lumbar interbody fusion. Eur Spine J 2011;20(4):612–7.

84. Garrett MP, Kakarla UK, Porter RW, et al. Formation of painful seroma and edema after the use of recombinant human bone morphogenetic protein-2 in posterolateral lumbar spine fusions. Neurosurgery 2010;66(6):1044–9 [discussion: 1049].

85. Ambrossi GL, McGirt MJ, Sciubba DM, et al. Recurrent lumbar disc herniation after single-level lumbar discectomy: incidence and health care cost analysis. Neurosurgery 2009;65(3):574–8 [discussion: 578].

86. Suk KS, Lee HM, Moon SH, et al. Recurrent lumbar disc herniation. Spine 2001;26(6):672–6.

87. Lee JK, Amorosa L, Cho SK, et al. Recurrent lumbar disk herniation. J Am Acad Orthop Surg 2010;18(6):327–37.

88. McGirt MJ, Eustacchio S, Varga P, et al. A prospective cohort study of close interval computed tomography and magnetic resonance imaging after primary lumbar discectomy: factors associated with recurrent disc herniation and disc height loss. Spine 2009;34(19):2044–51.

89. Lebow RL, Adogwa O, Parker SL, et al. Asymptomatic same-site recurrent disc herniation after lumbar discectomy: results of a prospective longitudinal study with 2-year serial imaging. Spine 2011;36(25):2147–51.

90. Bundschuh C, Modic M, Ross JS, et al. Epidural fibrosis and recurrent disk herniation in the lumbar spine: MR imaging assessment. AJR Am J Roentgenol 1988;150:923–32.

91. Ross JS. Magnetic resonance imaging of the postoperative spine. Semin Musculoskelet Radiol 2000;4(3):281–91.

92. Ross JS, Masaryk TJ, Schrader M, et al. MR imaging of the postoperative lumbar spine: assessment with gadopentetate dimeglumine. AJR Am J Roentgenol 1990;155(4):867–72.

93. Lawrence BD, Hilibrand AS, Brodt ED, et al. Predicting the risk of adjacent segment pathology in the cervical spine: a systematic review. Spine 2012;37(Suppl 22):S52–64.

94. Lawrence BD, Wang J, Arnold PM, et al. Predicting the risk of adjacent segment pathology after lumbar fusion. Spine 2012;37(Suppl 22):S123–32.

95. Lee MJ, Dettori JR, Standaert CJ, et al. The natural history of degeneration of the lumbar and cervical spines: a systematic review. Spine 2012;37(Suppl 22):S18–30.

96. Park P, Garton H, Gala V, et al. Adjacent segment disease after lumbar or lumbosacral

fusion: review of the literature. Spine 2004; 29(17):1938–44.

97. Kulkarni V, Rajshekhar V, Raghuram L. Accelerated spondylotic changes adjacent to the fused segment following central cervical corpectomy: magnetic resonance imaging study evidence. J Neurosurg 2004;100(1 Suppl Spine):2–6.

98. Anderson PA, Sasso RC, Hipp J, et al. Kinematics of the cervical adjacent segments after disc arthroplasty compared with anterior discectomy and fusion: a systematic review and meta-analysis. Spine 2012;37(Suppl 22):S85–95.

99. Khalatbari MR, Khalatbari I, Moharamzad Y. Intracranial hemorrhage following lumbar spine surgery. Eur Spine J 2012;21(10):2091–6.

100. Cevik B, Kirbas I, Cakir B, et al. Remote cerebellar hemorrhage after lumbar spinal surgery. Eur J Radiol 2009;70(1):7–9.

101. Konya D, Ozgen S, Pamir MN. Cerebellar hemorrhage after spinal surgery: case report and review of the literature. Eur Spine J 2006;15(1):95–9.

102. Baig MN, Lubow M, Immesoete P, et al. Vision loss after spine surgery: review of the literature and recommendations. Neurosurg Focus 2007;23(5):E15.

103. Lee LA, Newman NJ, Wagner TA, et al. Postoperative ischemic optic neuropathy. Spine 2010;35(9S): S105–16.

104. Al-Shafai L, Mikulis D. Diffusion MR imaging in a case of acute ischemic optic neuropathy. AJNR Am J Neuroradiol 2006;27:255–7.

Postoperative Spine Imaging in Cancer Patients

Esther E. Coronel, MD, Ruby J. Lien, MD,
A. Orlando Ortiz, MD, MBA*

KEYWORDS

- Postoperative spine • Spinal surgery • Spine tumors • Imaging • Complications • Spinal tumors
- Metastases

KEY POINTS

- Postoperative imaging of patients with spinal tumors plays a vital role in their management.
- Advances in magnetic resonance imaging, CT, and nuclear medicine have optimized postoperative imaging in patients with spinal cancer.
- Understanding of imaging protocols, expected postoperative findings, postoperative complications, and the appearance of tumor residual/recurrence is crucial for radiologists.

INTRODUCTION

Spine tumors can be classified according to their location in the spine: extradural, intradural extramedullary, and intramedullary. Metastatic spinal tumors are the most common type of malignant lesions of the spine, accounting for an estimated 70% of all spinal tumors. Common primary cancers that spread to the spine are lung, prostate, and breast cancer. The spine is the third most common site for metastatic disease and is the most common site for osseous metastases. Metastases to the spine can involve the bone, epidural space, spinal cord, and leptomeninges. Approximately 95% of metastatic spinal lesions are extradural in location, consisting of pure epidural lesions and lesions arising from the vertebral bodies, spreading to the epidural space.[1]

Most extradural tumors are metastatic, and the thoracic spine is the most commonly affected site. Multiple myeloma, lymphoma, and leukemia can also involve the spine and often present with multifocal or single-level extradural involvement. Primary malignant extradural tumors, such as osteosarcomas and Ewing sarcomas, are less common, as are primary nonmalignant entities, such

as osteoid osteomas and aneurysmal bone cysts. Management of extradural tumors includes gross total or subtotal surgical resection for surgical decompression with stabilization, chemotherapy, radiation therapy, and bone grafting.

Intradural extramedullary spread of systemic cancer comprises approximately 5% to 6% of spinal metastases.[1] Primary intradural extramedullary tumors comprise approximately 66% of all primary spinal tumors.[2] The most common intradural extramedullary tumors are schwannomas, followed by meningiomas. These tumors are usually slow-growing tumors that are treated by surgical resection only if patients exhibit significant neurologic symptoms caused by cord compression. The location of the tumor (ie, ventral or dorsal to the spinal cord) determines the operative approach: anterior, lateral, or posterior.

Intramedullary metastases are rare and comprise 0.5% to 1% of spinal metastases.[1] Primary intramedullary tumors include glial neoplasms, most commonly ependymomas and astrocytomas, and nonglial neoplasms, such as hemangioblastomas. These tumors are commonly treated with surgical resection. For ependymomas and astrocytomas, adjuvant radiation therapy may

Disclosures: None.
Department of Radiology, Winthrop-University Hospital, 259 First Street, Mineola, NY 11501, USA
* Corresponding author.
E-mail address: oortiz@winthrop.org

Neuroimag Clin N Am 24 (2014) 327–335
http://dx.doi.org/10.1016/j.nic.2014.01.009
1052-5149/14/$ – see front matter © 2014 Elsevier Inc. All rights reserved.

be used for lesions that undergo subtotal resection, and chemotherapy for failed radiation therapy or recurrence.

The treatment of spinal metastatic disease is multidisciplinary, dependent on patient presentation, and mostly palliative. Patients who present with pain without neurologic symptoms are treated primarily with site-directed radiation therapy and chemotherapy. Surgery is indicated for patients presenting with progressive neurologic deficits, neural compression due to retropulsed bone or epidural disease, spinal deformity or instability, and for treatment of radiation-resistant tumors.[3] A variety of surgical methods are available to treat metastatic disease to the spine. Dorsal spinal decompression and stabilization is the standard surgical technique to treat thoracic and lumbar metastases. Cervical metastases are treated with ventral decompression with corpectomy, vertebral body replacement, and ventral, stable-angle plate osteosynthesis.[4]

INDICATIONS FOR POSTOPERATIVE IMAGING

In the immediate postoperative period, imaging is performed to assess the extent of tumor resection. If surgical debulking of the tumor has been performed with the intention of subsequent radiation therapy or chemotherapy, an immediate follow-up magnetic resonance (MR) imaging is generally obtained to establish a baseline before therapy. Comparison with the preoperative imaging examination is a critical step in interpreting the postoperative study properly and in making distinctions between postoperative changes and the presence of residual neoplasm. Imaging evaluation is sometimes obtained on an emergent basis in symptomatic patients to assess for postsurgical complications. Common postsurgical complications in this patient population include hematoma, infection, ischemia, cerebrospinal fluid (CSF) leak, and malpositioning of hardware (Table 1).

Long-term routine follow-up imaging is obtained 4 to 6 months after surgery in the asymptomatic patient to assess for tumor recurrence or progression of disease. Long-term imaging is also obtained in the symptomatic patient to assess for hardware malpositioning or failure and to assess for treatment-related complications, such as radiation therapy–related vertebral compression fractures, radiation myositis, and radiation myelitis.

IMAGING PROTOCOLS
MR Imaging

Following tumor resection, postsurgical inflammation and neovascularity may develop within 24 hours, causing enhancement. Early MR imaging is therefore necessary to establish an accurate baseline, allowing the radiologist to distinguish between tumoral and postsurgical enhancement.

Due to the oftentimes subtle nature of tumoral enhancement and the difficulty in identifying it in the background of postsurgical scarring, postcontrast sequences must be performed with reliable fat saturation. Frequency-selective fat-saturation methods depend on the different resonance frequencies of water and fat. To suppress the fat signal accurately, the magnetic field must be homogeneous. This suppression is not possible in postoperative spines with hardware or metallic debris. Therefore, an alternative method of fat saturation with short tau inversion recovery (STIR) is preferred.[5] STIR imaging relies on the different relaxation times of tissues, using a 180° inversion pulse, allowing the longitudinal recovery of fat to reach a null point, and then applying a 90°

Table 1
Indications for postoperative imaging

Immediate	Routine	1. Assess extent of resection 2. Baseline for follow-up imaging (pre-RT and chemotherapy)
	Emergent/symptomatic	Assess for complications • Hematoma • Ischemia • Infection • CSF leak • Hardware failure/malposition
Long-term	Routine (4–6 mo) Emergent/symptomatic	Assess for tumor recurrence or progression 1. Assess for tumor recurrence 2. Assess for hardware failure 3. Assess for treatment-related effects (RT-VCF, myositis, myelitis)

Abbreviations: RT, radiation therapy; RT-VCF, radiation therapy-vertebral compression fractures.

radiofrequency pulse before echoing. However, STIR imaging also has its drawbacks, suffering from decreased signal-to-noise ratios, as well as increased scan times. Another method of obtaining fat suppression is achieved with the Dixon technique, which is a water-fat separation technique based on the different precessing velocities of water and fat. The Dixon method was previously hampered by field inhomogeneities. However, new variants, including the iterative decomposition of water and fat with echo asymmetry and least-squares estimation, have shown promise in separating water and fat while taking into account field inhomogeneities, resulting in optimal, uniform fat suppression with high signal-to-noise ratio and image quality.[6]

Another challenge in imaging the postoperative spine is the susceptibility artifact caused by metallic hardware, which results in signal loss and geometric distortion, which can be compensated by thinner slices, smaller voxels, and excessive radiofrequency refocusing. New techniques using 3D volumetric fast spin-echo imaging are now used with isotropic voxels, which provide high signal-to-noise ratio and spatial resolution, with relatively short scan times, using parallel imaging and phased array coils and sequences obtained with long echo train lengths. Resultant blurring is compensated for by flip angle modulations during readout (CUBE, Volumetric ISotropic T2-weighted Acquisition, Sampling Perfection with Application optimized Contrasts using flip-angle Evolutions).[7]

In addition, diffusion-weighted imaging (DWI) has been found to be a helpful adjunct to traditional sequences in spine imaging and may be particularly useful for postoperative tumor surveillance patients. DWI offers unique information on tissue characteristics by reflecting the motion of water molecules in tissues. In the initial postoperative period, fluid collections may be characterized with DWI. Abscesses with pus will generally demonstrate high signal on DWI with reduced apparent diffusion coefficient, whereas seromas will not. Furthermore, there has been research suggesting the utility of DWI in patients with osseous metastases. In the differentiation of acute benign osteoporotic compression fractures from pathologic compression fractures, T1 and T2 sequences are inadequate, often demonstrating similar signal intensities in both conditions. DWI has proven helpful in this distinction with hyperintense signal in acute pathologic compression fractures and hypointense signal in acute benign fractures.[8] However, research on the utility of DWI in detecting vertebral metastases have yielded varying results with some studies demonstrating that it does not surpass traditional T1-weighted sequences and others demonstrating an advantage to adding the DWI sequence.[9] Although more studies need to be performed on the use of DWI in the follow-up of treated vertebral metastases, there have been several small studies suggesting their usefulness with decreased signal intensity in lesions that have undergone successful therapy.[10]

Computed Tomography

Computed tomography (CT) is the preferred imaging modality to evaluate spinal hardware for malpositioning and fracture. However, the metallic hardware produces significant artifact on CT. When spinal fixation hardware is present, imaging parameters should be optimized to minimize artifact. Imaging techniques, including dual-energy CT, are now available to minimize many of these artifacts and are discussed elsewhere in this issue.

Nuclear Medicine

Common indications for nuclear medicine in assessing the postoperative spine include spinal infection, pseudoarthrosis, and recurrence or progression of tumors. Radionuclides that can be used to diagnose spinal infections include [99]Technetium[m]-methylene diphosphonate, single-photon emission computed tomography (SPECT), 3-phase bone, [67]Gallium citrate, [111]Indium oxine–labeled leukocytes, and 18-F-fluoro-deoxy-D-glucose (FDG)-labeled positron emission tomographic (PET) scans.

With the advent of new cancer therapies, patients with metastatic disease are demonstrating longer lifespans than before, and new imaging modalities are needed to monitor vertebral metastases. Spinal FDG-PET/CT has demonstrated accuracy in the detection of metastases with increased tracer uptake reflecting the increased glucose metabolism in lesions.[11–13] More importantly, it is becoming an emerging modality in assisting radiation therapy planning following surgical debulking due to its ability to delineate lesions despite overlying hardware.[14] It has also been shown to monitor response to therapy effectively.[15,16] Continued research is being performed with various radionuclides for PET imaging with increased specificity for certain cancers and seems promising.

IMAGING FINDINGS

In the immediate postoperative period, MR imaging is obtained to assess for the extent of resection and residual malignancy. The MR imaging is done within 24 hours following surgery before neovascularity and scarring develop. Any significant enhancing tissue can therefore be more reliably determined to be residual tumor. Common postoperative changes, including muscle edema, paraspinal seromas, and trace hemorrhage, should be expected (**Fig. 1**).

Imaging may also be obtained on an emergent basis in the immediate postoperative period in symptomatic patients to assess for postsurgical complications, such as hematoma, infection, ischemia, CSF leak, and malpositioning of hardware. Symptomatic spinal epidural hematomas are an infrequent complication of spinal surgery. They typically occur within the first 24 hours following surgery and very rarely occur up to 1 week after surgery.[17] MR imaging demonstrates a biconcave, elongated mass in the epidural space with variable degrees of cord compression. The signal intensity of the hematoma varies depending on the age of the hemorrhage.

The incidence of surgical site infections in adult spine surgeries ranges from 0.7% to 20% and varies with the type of surgery. A posterior surgical approach and the utilization of spinal hardware carry an increased risk of infection.[18] Studies have also demonstrated a higher incidence of wound infections in patients who have been treated with radiation before surgery.[19] Postoperative infections may occur early, within 1 month of surgery, or may be delayed and occur 3 to 9 months after surgery.[18] They range from superficial skin incision infections to deep-tissue infections and include infected seromas, paraspinal abscesses, and/or osteomyelitis/discitis.[20] The appearance of these entities on MR imaging has been described in detail elsewhere in this issue. In cases where MR imaging cannot be performed or is nondiagnostic due to metallic artifact, bone scintigraphy including SPECT combined with radionuclide-labeled white blood cells can be helpful in the detection of infection.[21]

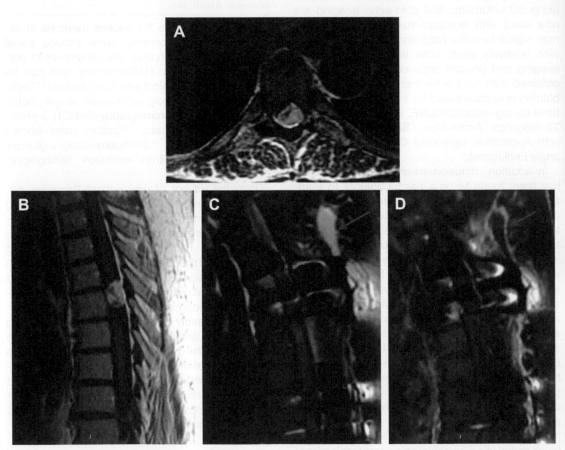

Fig. 1. A 52-year-old woman with a history of schwannoma in the upper thoracic spine. Contrast-enhanced T1-weighted axial (*A*) and sagittal (*B*) images show an enhancing intradural extramedullary mass that compresses the spinal cord. The patient was treated with surgical resection with laminectomy and fixation. Immediate postoperative study demonstrates seroma (*arrow*) in the paraspinal soft tissues on sagittal STIR image (*C*) and T1 fat-saturated post-gadolinium image (*D*).

In patients who have had spinal instrumentation, hardware malpositioning and fracture can be seen in both the early and the late postoperative stages. Hardware positioning and integrity are best evaluated on CT. Various components of the hardware can be malpositioned or fractured (**Figs. 2** and **3**). Various types of pedicle screws are commonly used today and optimal screw placement is typically along the medial aspect of the pedicle. Common complications of pedicle screws include penetration of the anterior cortex and fracture of the screws. Loosening of pedicle screws may often be seen as lucency around the screw threads that exceed 2 mm or increase in size.[11,21]

Another late complication of spinal instrumentation is pseudoarthrosis. Bone grafting is commonly used in conjunction with spinal instrumentation procedures. Normal fusion is usually identified radiographically 6 to 9 months after the procedure. In the presence of chronic low-grade instability and motion, pseudoarthrosis may develop, which results from fibrous union of the fusion complex, instead of osseous union. Pseudoarthrosis has

been reported in 15% to 20% of patients and usually manifests months to years after the initial operation.[22–24] Patients commonly present with axial or radicular pain. Mature pseudoarthrosis typically presents as linear lucency through the bone graft. Early pseudoarthrosis may have a more subtle appearance on CT, and radionuclide bone scans may be helpful in confirming the diagnosis. Bone scans may remain positive for a year or more in the region of the graft, demonstrating ill-defined or diffuse activity due to continued bone remodeling at the fusion site. However, very focal intense activity suggests pseudoarthrosis.[11,24] MR imaging is also sensitive for evaluating pseudoarthrosis. T2-weighted images demonstrate focal high-signal intensity in the region of pseudoarthrosis with corresponding bands of low intensity on T1-weighted images.[11,21]

In addition to assessing for complications related to hardware, long-term imaging is also obtained in the symptomatic patient to assess for treatment-related effects, such as radiation therapy–related vertebral compression fractures,

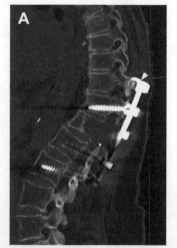

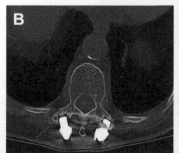
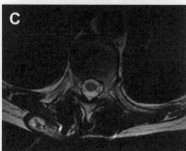
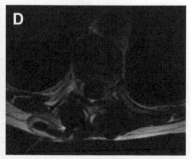

Fig. 2. A 75-year-old woman with a history of hemangioendothelioma of the thoracic spine treated with corpectomy and stabilization. Follow-up imaging for back pain demonstrates malpositioning of stabilization hardware with the superior T8 transverse process hook posteriorly positioned (*arrow*) (*A, B*). Subsequent MR imaging of the thoracic spine shows a fluid collection surrounding the hook on the T2-weighted axial image (*arrow*) (*C*) with an enhancing margin (*arrow*) seen on the T1 post-gadolinium image (*D*), consistent with irritation of the paraspinal soft tissues and bursa formation.

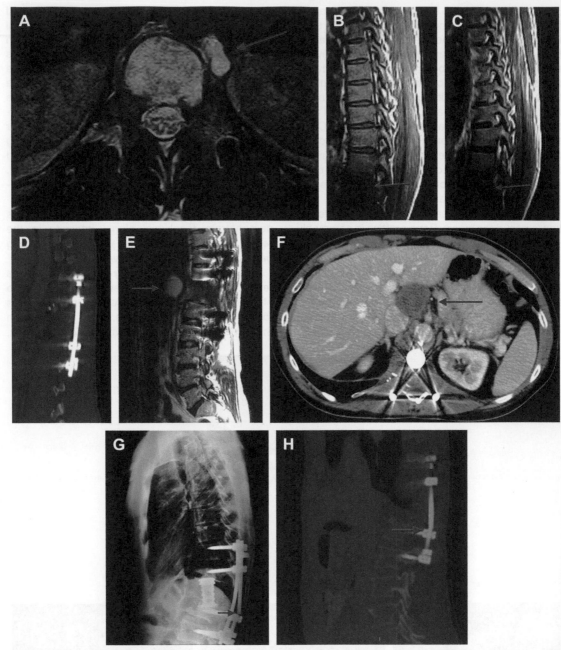

Fig. 3. A 53-year-old man with a remote history of resected liposarcoma of the ankle presents with back pain. T2-weighted axial MR image shows a T12 vertebral body metastasis with an anterior paraspinal soft tissue component on T2 (*arrow*) (*A*). T1 pre- and postcontrast images (*B, C*) show that the lesion is hypointense with minimal peripheral enhancement (*arrow*). The patient was treated with lesion resection and corpectomy and stabilized anteriorly and posteriorly. Immediate follow-up sagittal CT reformation shows intact hardware (*D*). One year later, a new lesion (*arrow*) was detected anterior to the surgical site as shown on the T2 sagittal MR image (*E*); a contrast-enhanced CT of the abdomen shows that this mass is located in the porta hepatis (*arrow*) (*F*). The lesion was treated with Cyberknife radiosurgery, which facilitated subsequent resection. A 1-year follow-up plain radiograph (*G*) and sagittal CT reformation (*H*) show a fracture (*arrow*) of the fixation rod.

radiation myositis, and radiation myelopathy. Characteristic findings of radiation myositis on MR include edema throughout the radiation field and straight, sharp margins of edema that extend across muscle and subcutaneous fat.[24] Radiation myelopathy is a rare and late complication of radiation therapy that is usually seen within 4 years after radiation treatment. The incidence depends on the total radiation dose, dose per fraction, and length of spinal cord irradiated. With the conventionally fractionated doses, a total dose of approximately 57 to 61 Gy has been correlated to a 5% incidence of radiation myelopathy, and a total dose of 68 to 73 Gy has been correlated to a 50% incidence.[25,26] The MR imaging appearance of radiation myelopathy varies and does not correlate with patients' onset or severity of symptoms. Early in the course, less than 8 months after symptom onset, MR imaging may demonstrate a combination of low T1 and high T2 signal, cord swelling, and enhancement. In the later stages, 3 years after the onset of symptoms, MR imaging generally demonstrates cord atrophy.[25] Additional findings of adjacent hyperintense vertebral bodies on T2-weighted images suggest prior radiation treatment.[27]

Routine long-term follow-up imaging is often obtained 4 to 6 months after surgery to assess for tumor recurrence or progression of disease (Fig. 4). Spinal metastases have a higher recurrence rate compared with primary spinal tumors. The risk of recurrent metastatic disease is highest if wide or total resection is not achieved and if irradiation precedes surgery.[28] Intramedullary tumors such as ependymomas have a 10-year recurrence rate of 5.1%, whereas more aggressive, infiltrating tumors such as astrocytomas have a 10-year recurrence rate of 40.9%.[29] MR imaging is the imaging modality of choice to assess for recurrent malignancy (see Fig. 4). Vertebral metastases demonstrate low signal on T1, usually with associated enhancement, and epidural metastases will present as enhancing soft tissue. Recurrent primary spine tumors will also demonstrate enhancing soft tissue, not present on the immediate postoperative scans (Fig. 5). FDG-PET is a useful adjunct in determining therapeutic response to radiation therapy and chemotherapy.[12] Many

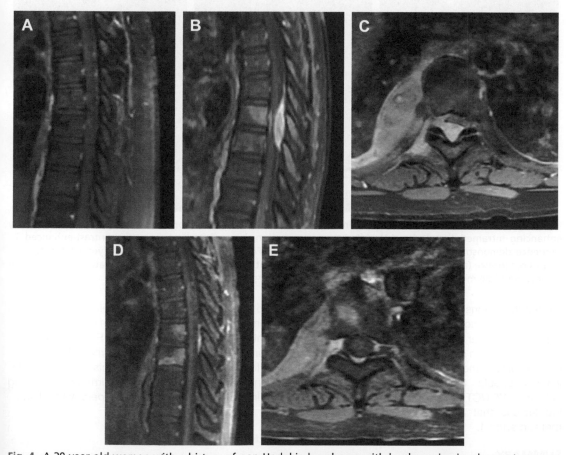

Fig. 4. A 39-year-old woman with a history of non-Hodgkin lymphoma with lumbar spine involvement was successfully treated with chemotherapy and radiation therapy. Follow-up study 4 years following treatment demonstrates no evidence of thoracic spine involvement (A) on this fat-saturated T1 post-gadolinium image. Patient then developed new-onset mid back pain 4 years later (B, C), with new osseous and epidural metastases at T8–T9 resulting in severe cord compression and extension to the right pleura. Following radiation therapy (D, E), the patient demonstrated significant improvement.

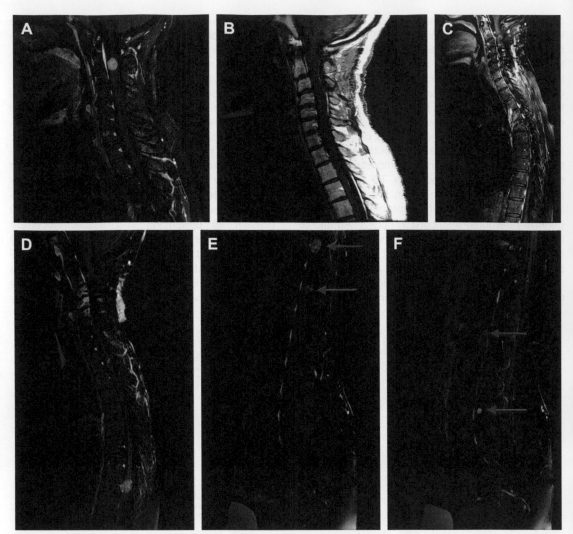

Fig. 5. A patient with cervical ependymoma. Postcontrast T1 image demonstrates well-circumscribed avidly enhancing intramedullary lesion (A). After surgical resection, immediate postoperative contrast-enhanced T1 sequence demonstrates no evidence of residual tumor (B). Follow-up surveillance study 3 years later demonstrates recurrence (arrows) at C2 and C3 levels (C). The patient developed back pain 2 years later and was found to have multiple metastatic lesions (arrows) throughout the spine (D–F).

metastatic lesions demonstrate increased activity following radiation or chemotherapy due to increased cellular turnover, reflecting a response to therapy known as the flare phenomenon, which can last up to 6 months, at which point responding lesions should then demonstrate decreased activity.[30] PET/CT is particularly helpful in detecting lesions that may be obscured on MR by metallic artifact.

SUMMARY

The paradigm of managing patients with spinal tumors has significantly changed in recent years because of the development of new cancer therapies. Patients' life expectancies are being prolonged, and the focus on their care has shifted from palliation to the treatment of residual or recurrent tumor and complications. Postoperative imaging, therefore, plays a more vital role than ever before in the management of this patient population. Radiologists must have a firm understanding of imaging protocols and postoperative findings.

REFERENCES

1. Sham LM, Salzman KL. Imaging of spinal metastatic disease. Int J Surg Oncol 2011;1–12.
2. Ahn D, Park H, Choi D, et al. The surgical treatment for spinal intradural extramedullary tumors. Clin Orthop Surg 2009;1(3):165–72.

3. Singh K, Samartzis D, Vacarro AR, et al. Current concepts in the management of metastatic spinal disease. J Bone Joint Surg Br 2006;4:434–42.

4. Delank KS, Wendtner C, Eich HT, et al. The treatment of spinal metastases. Dtsch Arztebl Int 2011; 108(5):71–80.

5. Stradiotti P, Curti A, Castellazzi G, et al. Metal-related artifacts in instrumented spine. Techniques for reducing artifacts in CT and MRI: state of the art. Eur Spine J 2009;18(Suppl 1):S102–8.

6. Ren AJ, Guo Y, Tian SP, et al. MR imaging of the spine at 3.0 T with T2-weighted IDEAL fast recovery fast spin-echo technique. Korean J Radiol 2012; 13(1):44–52.

7. Lighvani AA, Melhem ER. Advances in high-field MR imaging of the spine. Appl Radiol 2009;6:18–27.

8. Baur A, Stabler A, Bruning R, et al. Diffusion-weighted MR imaging of bone marrow: differentiation of benign versus pathologic compression fractures. Radiology 1998;207:349–56.

9. Castillo M, Arbelaez A, Smith JK, et al. Diffusion-weighted MR imaging offers no advantage over routine noncontrast MR imaging in the detection of vertebral metastases. AJNR Am J Neuroradiol 2000;21:948–53.

10. Byun WM, Shin SO, Chang Y, et al. Diffusion-weighted MR imaging of metastatic disease of the spine: assessment of response to therapy. AJNR Am J Neuroradiol 2002;23:906–12.

11. Nouh MR. Spinal fusion-hardware construct: basic concepts and imaging review. World J Radiol 2012;4(5):193–207.

12. Sandu N, Popperl G, Toubert M, et al. Current molecular imaging of spinal tumors in clinical practice. Mol Med 2011;17(3–4):308–16.

13. Wieser E, Skripkus UJ, Wang J. The role of nuclear medicine imaging in the diagnosis and management of postoperative spinal infections in the setting of instrumentation. Semin Spine Surg 2004;16(3):156–61.

14. Gwak HS, Youn SM, Chang U, et al. Usefulness of (18)F-fluorodeoxyglucose PET for radiosurgery planning and response monitoring in patients with recurrent spinal metastasis. Minim Invasive Neurosurg 2006;49(3):127–34.

15. Laufer I, Lis E, Pisinski L, et al. The accuracy of 18F-fluorodeoxyglucose positron emission tomography as confirmed by biopsy in the diagnosis of spine metastases in a cancer population. Neurosurgery 2009;64(1):107–14.

16. De Geus-Oei LF, Vriens D, van Laarhoven HW, et al. Monitoring and predicting response to therapy with 18F-FDG PET in colorectal cancer: a systemic review. J Nucl Med 2009;50:43S–54S.

17. Amiri AR, Fouyas IP, Cro S, et al. Postoperative spinal epidural hematoma (SEH): incidence, risk factors, onset, and management. Spine J 2013;13(2): 134–40.

18. Gerometta A, Olaverri JC, Bitan F. Infections in spinal instrumentation. Int Orthop 2012;38(2): 457–64.

19. Ghogawala Z, Mansfield FL, Borges LF. Spinal radiation before surgical decompression adversely affects outcomes of surgery for symptomatic metastatic spinal cord compression. Spine 2001;26: 818–24.

20. Sasso RC, Garrido BJ. Postoperative spinal wound infections. J Am Acad Orthop Surg 2008;16(6): 330–7.

21. Young PM, Berquist TH, Bancroft LW, et al. Complications of spinal instrumentation. Radiographics 2007;27:775–89.

22. Berquist TH. Imaging of the post-operative spine. Radiol Clin North Am 2006;44:407–18.

23. Raizman NM, O'Brien JR, Peohling-Monaghan KL, et al. Pseudoarthrosis of the spine. J Am Acad Orthop Surg 2009;17(8):494–503.

24. May DA, Disler DG, Jones EA, et al. Abnormal signal intensity in skeletal muscle at MR imaging: patterns, pearls, and pitfalls. Radiographics 2000; 20:S295–315.

25. Naidich TP, Castillo M, Raybaud C, et al. Imaging of the spine: expert radiology series, expert consult. Philadelphia: Saunders/Elsevier; 2011. p. 489–90.

26. Gocheva L. Radiation tolerance of the spinal cord: doctrine, dogmas, data. Arch Oncol 2000;8(3): 131–4.

27. Jacob A, Weinshenker BG. An approach to the diagnosis of acute transverse myelitis. Semin Neurol 2008;28(1):105–20.

28. Van der Sande JJ, Boogerd W, Kroger R, et al. Recurrent spinal epidural metastases: a prospective study with a complete follow up. J Neurol Neurosurg Psychiatry 1999;66(5):623–7.

29. Klekamp J. Treatment of intramedullary tumors: analysis of surgical morbidity and long-term results. J Neurosurg Spine 2013;19:12–26.

30. Wade AA, Scott JA, Kuter I, et al. Flare response in 18F-fluoride ion PET bone scanning. AJR Am J Roentgenol 2006;186:1783–6.

Post-Vertebral Augmentation Spine Imaging

Sudhir Kathuria, MD

KEYWORDS

• Vertebral augmentation • Cement leakage • Compression fracture • Post vertebroplasty imaging

KEY POINTS

- The goal of the vertebral augmentation (VA) procedure is to relieve pain by providing structural stability of the fractured vertebra through the safe injection of a stabilizing material.
- Complications from VA procedures are rare and generally result from unrecognized leakage of acrylic bone cement. Meticulous needle-placement technique and fluoroscopic monitoring during careful cement injection contribute to the safe performance of these procedures.
- Any worsening of the clinical symptoms during or after the VA procedure should warrant an urgent computed tomography (CT) scan to assess for potential cement leak.
- A new neurologic deficit should lead to an emergent CT scan and spine surgical consult.
- It is important to be aware of the expected imaging changes in previously augmented vertebrae.
- Magnetic resonance imaging should be strongly considered in the evaluation of patients presenting with unexplained new or residual symptoms after an initial successful VA procedure.
- Persistent edema and interval height loss after a successful VA procedure should not be interpreted as sufficient evidence of ongoing abnormality at the treated vertebral level.
- To make an accurate diagnosis, it is of vital importance to apply the knowledge of expected imaging changes in treated vertebrae, and correlate post-VA imaging findings with new clinical symptoms and the physical examination.

INTRODUCTION

The osteoporotic population at risk of compression fracture is sizable, with more than 700,000 new fractures every year in the United States alone.[1] Although imaging plays a critical role and has become an integral part in preprocedure evaluation of these patients, a substantial number of treated patients undergo follow-up imaging. Reasons for obtaining follow-up imaging range from potential procedure-related complications to development of new symptoms after initial improvement from a successful vertebral augmentation (VA). Although imaging is frequently obtained for evaluation of these patients, there is a general lack of knowledge about imaging characteristics of treated vertebrae. This article reviews

various indications for post-VA imaging, the appearance of augmented spine on imaging; especially magnetic resonance (MR) imaging, and the important complications associated with the VA procedure.

VERTEBRAL AUGMENTATION

VA is a percutaneous, imaged-guided procedure primarily used for treating back pain associated with vertebral compression fractures that are not effectively treated by conservative or medical therapy.[2,3] This procedure was first introduced as a technique for the treatment of a symptomatic cervical vertebral hemangioma in 1987.[2] Since then, it has become a valuable and frequently used therapeutic option in the management of back pain

The Russell H. Morgan Department of Radiology and Radiological Science, Johns Hopkins Hospital, 1800 Orleans Street, Bloomberg 7218, Baltimore, MD 21287, USA
E-mail address: skathur2@jhmi.edu

Neuroimag Clin N Am 24 (2014) 337–347
http://dx.doi.org/10.1016/j.nic.2014.01.007

caused by osteoporotic and pathologic vertebral compression fractures.

The fundamental aim of the VA procedure is to improve pain, stability, and compressive strength of the vertebral body through the safe injection of a stabilizing material. This goal can be achieved by both vertebroplasty and kyphoplasty. Vertebroplasty involves the injection of acrylic bone cement inside the fractured vertebra using a needle under image guidance, generally x-ray or computed tomography (CT) fluoroscopy. Kyphoplasty, in comparison with vertebroplasty, involves the additional step of creating a cavity inside the diseased vertebral body by temporarily inflating a balloon tamp followed by injection of the bone cement into the cavity.

The usefulness of cross-sectional imaging in preprocedure evaluation of a VA procedure, including MR imaging and CT, is well established.[4] MR imaging provides information on anatomic vertebral collapse and marrow edema that is essential for identifying the location and extent of the disease (Fig. 1). It also provides useful information about any canal or neural compromise. CT is helpful in identifying the potential route of cement extravasations by demonstrating any open fracture lines and osseous destruction, especially in pathologic fractures.[5]

By contrast, the indications and role of imaging in the post-VA setting is not as well described, but is becoming increasingly important.

REASONS FOR POST-VA IMAGING

Reasons for obtaining post-VA imaging can be broadly categorized as shown in Box 1.

Post-VA Baseline Imaging

Single or biplane x-ray fluoroscopy has been the most widely used modality to perform VA procedures. Radiographic images in 2 orthogonal planes should be obtained at the end of each augmentation procedure for documentation and evaluation of cement distribution; this is generally sufficient for an uneventful treatment of an osteoporotic vertebral compression fracture. Routine postprocedure CT imaging should be considered after treatment of pathologic vertebral fractures. There is increasing use of CT fluoroscopy to perform VA procedures in both osteoporotic and pathologic compression fractures. In such cases, CT images are obtained at the completion of the procedure. This CT scan provides useful baseline information about the distribution of acrylic bone cement and also demonstrates any unsuspected complications including cement leakage, changes

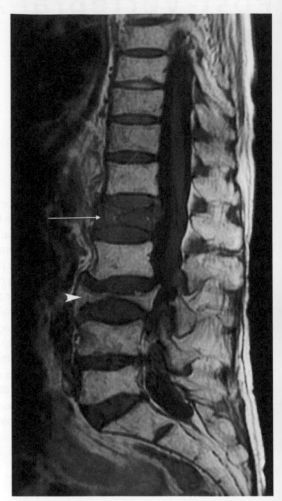

Fig. 1. T1-weighted magnetic resonance (MR) image shows the acute nature of L1 vertebral compression fracture by demonstrating edema as low signal intensity (*arrow*). Compare this with the L3 vertebral compression fracture with no edema, suggesting its chronic nature (*arrowhead*). Only the L1 level was treated with vertebral augmentation (VA), with complete resolution of the patient's symptoms of back pain.

Box 1
Categories of reasons for obtaining post-VA

1. Baseline imaging obtained at the completion of an uneventful procedure

2. Imaging obtained for further evaluation of suspected complications resulting from the augmentation procedure

3. Imaging obtained for evaluation of new or recurrent symptoms after initial improvement

in tumor position, procedure-related hematoma, and fracture.[5]

Post-VA Imaging for Suspected Complications

Fortunately, the complication rate with VA procedures is low and ranges from 1.3% for osteoporosis, to 2.5% for hemangiomas, and 10% for neoplastic disease.[5] The commonly encountered complications during VA are further discussed here.

Cement leakage

Cement leakage accounts for most symptomatic complications that can occur in association with VA. The primary cause is the leakage of acrylic bone cement beyond the confines of the vertebral body into the epidural and/or paravertebral venous plexus (Fig. 2) or into adjacent spaces via existing fracture lines and cortical destruction. Cement leaks may be seen in up to 15% of routine cases. The overwhelming majority of these leaks is generally small and of no clinical significance.[6]

Any acute worsening of the patient's clinical symptoms during or immediately after the procedure should warrant a CT scan to assess the size and location of potential cement extravasation.

A new neurologic deficit should lead to an immediate CT scan and possible spine surgical consultation. The most common consequence of a symptomatic cement leakage occurs locally, producing radiculopathy from nerve-root irritation or myelopathy from cord compression. Nerve-root irritation may be transient, and is treatable with nonsteroidal anti-inflammatory medications or local steroid injections (Fig. 3). Persistent pain may require surgical removal of the extravasated cement. Cord compression may result in paresis or paralysis, and requires immediate surgical intervention. In one series of 40 patients with osteolytic metastases or myeloma, venous and cortical cement leaks were identified in 29 of 40 patients using post-procedure CT scans.[7] Most of these cement leaks were asymptomatic, but 2 of 8 foraminal cement leaks produced nerve-root compression that required decompressive surgery. In another subsequent series, only 3 of 13 patients with radicular pain required surgical treatments while another 10 responded well to local anesthetic infiltration or medical therapy.[8] Only 1 of 258 treated patients experienced spinal cord compression that required surgery.[8]

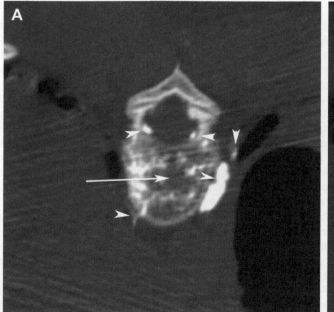
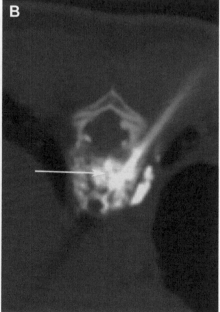

Fig. 2. A middle-aged woman presented with a symptomatic vertebral body hemangioma. The patient underwent x-ray fluoroscopy–guided vertebroplasty at another institution and presented for a second opinion. (A) Postvertebroplasty computed tomography (CT) image shows several areas of asymptomatic cement leakage into venous structures outside of the vertebral body (multiple *arrowheads*). Note that there was no cement filling inside the hemangioma (*arrow* indicates center of hemangioma). She still had her original symptoms of back pain with no new symptoms from leakage. (B) A repeat vertebroplasty procedure was performed under CT guidance. Note the needle in place with cement filling inside the hemangioma (*arrow*). Her symptoms improved significantly after this procedure.

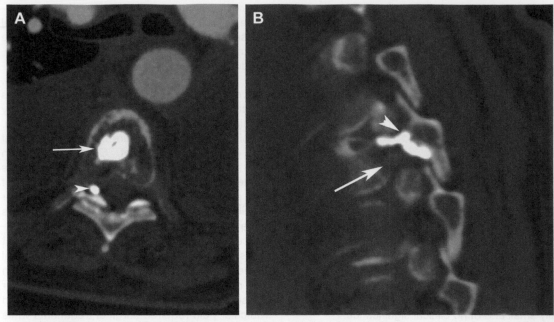

Fig. 3. Asymptomatic neural foraminal cement leakage during VA of a pathologic compression fracture. (*A*) Axial CT image demonstrates hyperdense cement inside the treated vertebral body (*arrow*). Note the small separate focus of cement (*arrowhead*) along the neural foramen that was identified during the cement injection; further cement injection was immediately stopped. (*B*) Reformatted sagittal CT image in the same patient better demonstrates the cement leakage (*arrowhead*) tracking adjacent to, but not impinging on, the nerve root (*arrow*).

Another common location for cement leakage is intravasation into venous structures. Migration of small amounts of acrylic bone cement to the pulmonary veins is generally without clinical significance, but symptomatic pulmonary embolus (**Fig. 4**) and death have been reported.[5] In otherwise healthy individuals, the lungs can tolerate small acrylic cement emboli without symptoms. However, a large cement bolus can cause pulmonary infarct, and multiple emboli may lead to pulmonary compromise or even death.[9] An operator can take 2 important steps to diagnose this complication. First, it is necessary to monitor the patient's vital signs and oxygen saturation before, during, and after the VA procedure. Any sudden and unexplained alteration of the patient's respiratory rate, heart rate, or oxygen saturation should raise the possibility of a potential acute pulmonary embolic event. Second, careful periprocedural fluoroscopic monitoring will help the operator to detect cement extravasation and, therefore, stop the cement injection. Chest radiographs and/or CT of the thorax may be required to confirm the presence of cement emboli.

New fractures following VA often occur, and may reflect the natural history of osteoporosis rather than a complication of the procedure.

However, several studies have shown an increased risk of developing adjacent-level fractures following the leakage of acrylic bone cement into the disc space.[10] These results should be considered with caution, as adjacent-level fractures after VA are also known to occur without any intradiscal leakage.[11] Recent data from the VERTOS II trial, which randomized painful vertebral compression fractures to either treatment with conservative management or VA, showed no significant increased incidence of new compression fractures in patients who had cement leakage into the disc at 12 months' follow-up.[12] The only risk factor identified in this study for a new vertebral compression fracture was the number of baseline vertebral compression fractures; patients with multiple vertebral compression fractures at presentation were at increased risk of developing a subsequent vertebral compression within a year after presentation. A small amount of cement extravasation into the disc may not be of consequence, but the authors suggest that all precautions should be taken to avoid any significant leakage of acrylic bone cement into the disc (**Fig. 5**). A meta-analysis of the VA literature shows that the subsequent fracture rate for VA procedures (11%) is one-half that of patients who undergo nonsurgical management (22%).[13]

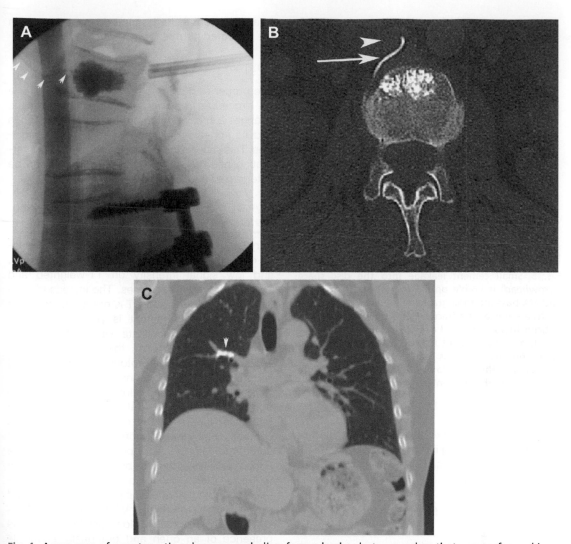

Fig. 4. A rare case of symptomatic pulmonary embolism from a kyphoplasty procedure that was performed in an operating room. (*A*) Lateral fluoroscopic image at the end of the procedure shows a linear radiopaque density (path marked by multiple *arrowheads*) that follows the course of a paraspinal vein; this was not initially noticed during cement injection. Change in the patient's oxygen saturation led to an urgent CT scan. (*B*) Axial CT image at the level of the VA procedure clearly demonstrates the linear extraosseous venous leakage of the cement (*arrow*) that enters into the inferior vena cava (*arrowhead*). (*C*) Coronal reconstruction of the chest CT confirming a cement embolus (*arrowhead*) into a right pulmonary artery branch.

Pain exacerbation

An idiopathic pain increase following VA is uncommon. Substantial local cement leaks may result in local pain exacerbation.[14] A CT scan through the treated spine segment should be immediately obtained to evaluate for any mechanical causes such as nerve-root or spinal cord impingement from cement leakage. If the CT examination shows no cement leakage or any other abnormality, the pain can be expected to be self-limiting and is likely to improve within a few hours.

Iatrogenic injury, infection, and bleeding

VA-related iatrogenic injury to vascular or neural structures can result from improper needle technique and positioning. Other rare complications that may occur during or following VA include iatrogenic fracture, infection, hematoma, and pneumothorax.[10]

Complications are best avoided by awareness of the factors that contribute to their occurrence. Following a meticulous technique for needle placement, meticulous fluoroscopic monitoring,

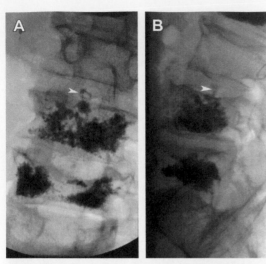

Fig. 5. Small cement leakage into the disc space (*arrowhead*) is visible on (*A*) frontal and (*B*) lateral post-VA baseline radiographs obtained after successful treatment of the fracture. This small leakage was noticed toward the end of the injection into the L4 vertebral body. Cement injection was stopped soon after the leakage was noticed to avoid further leakage into the disc. No new adjacent-level fracture was seen in this patient for up to 18 months of follow-up.

and avoidance of excessive pressure and/or cement volume during injection, especially after a small cement leakage has already been identified, is strongly suggested.

Post-VA Imaging for Evaluation of New Symptoms

It is relatively common for patients to present with renewed back pain at some time in the future after initial successful VA. This pain may be the result of a new compression fracture or other disorders such as facet arthritis, disc herniation, infection, central canal stenosis, and myofascial pain.[15,16] Although MR imaging is frequently obtained for evaluation of these patients, there is general lack of knowledge about the imaging characteristics of treated vertebrae. Radiologists and treating physicians often are confused and remain uncertain if the previously treated level is still contributing to the patient's symptoms of back pain. For accurate diagnosis, it is important to be aware of the expected imaging changes in previously augmented vertebrae. A limited number of published studies describe the normal imaging appearance of the post-VA spine.[15,17,18]

Based on this limited literature and the authors' own experience, the next section describes the spectrum of imaging findings in successfully treated vertebrae that can be considered within the expected normal range.[15,17,18]

POST-VA IMAGING APPEARANCE

The proper evaluation of a new back pain after a VA procedure requires an understanding of the changes a successful treated vertebra undergoes and its appearance on different imaging modalities. This knowledge is important in correctly interpreting post-VA images. These changes can be categorized into 3 main components (**Box 2**).

Signal Changes Resulting from the Cement Material

Acrylic bone cement produces hyperdense opacity on radiographs, increased attenuation on CT, and low signal intensity on T1-weighted and T2-weighted MR sequences. The increased density on radiography and CT is due to the fact that the acrylic bone cement is preopacified with barium sulfate to facilitate visualization during fluoroscopic injection. As this is essentially an implant with no mobile protons, absence of signal is detected with MR imaging.

The cement distribution pattern can be described as 2 main patterns: cleft type and trabecular type.[19] In the cleft type pattern, the cement distribution is more solid and compact compared with the more permeative sponge-like appearance in the trabecular type pattern (**Fig. 6**). A cleft indicates a cavity within the fractured vertebra that could be preexisting or created during a cavity-producing VA procedure such as kyphoplasty. Because of low resistance and the presence of an open and potentially expansile space, acrylic bone cement is generally easier to inject into the cleft, so the volume of cement injected tends to be greater for this type of distribution pattern. The degree of vertebral height gain after VA has also been shown to be greater for this pattern than with the trabecular pattern.[19] However, the distribution pattern seems to have no significant effect on the initial clinical response. It is not uncommon to find some combination of

---

Box 2
Categories of changes undergone by a successfully treated vertebra

1. Signal changes from cement material

2. Signal changes in bone marrow surrounding the cement material

3. Vertebral size and morphology changes resulting from cement injection

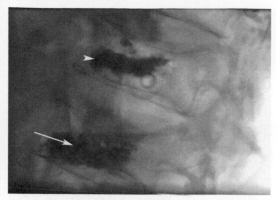

Fig. 6. Post-VA lateral radiograph of 2 treated fractures demonstrating 2 common types of cement-distribution pattern. Note the more cohesive cement filling in the cleft type pattern (*arrowhead*) at the upper level, versus the more permeative sponge-like distribution in the trabecular pattern (*arrow*) at the lower level.

both cement distribution patterns within the same treated vertebra.

Signal Changes in Bone Marrow Surrounding Cement Material

There is little known about the natural history of bone marrow edema on MR imaging in untreated vertebral compression fractures. Depending on the age of the fracture, MR imaging can show characteristic changes in the signal intensity of bone marrow. Acute or subacute fractures are manifested by low signal intensity on T1-weighted images and high signal intensity on T2-weighted and short-tau inversion recovery (STIR) sequences.[20] Bone marrow edema presumably results from microfractures of the trabeculae within the medullary bone. Studies have shown a positive correlation between the amount of edema and the degree of pain relief after a VA procedure, supporting the idea that the presence of bone marrow edema can be a useful supportive tool in selecting the vertebra to be treated.[3]

Although the presence of bone marrow edema in a fractured vertebra on pre-VA MR imaging is considered to be related to the painful level, little is known about the relationship of bone marrow edema with pain after a successful VA procedure. Studies have shown that while significant pain improvement happens within 3 months after VA, the bone marrow edema can persist, or even progress at times, with no associated pain.[17] Therefore, the presence of bone marrow edema on post-VA MR imaging should not be equated to ongoing pain at the treated vertebral level (**Fig. 7**). Temporal changes in post-VA bone

marrow edema on MR imaging can be categorized as early, intermediate, or late (**Box 3**).

Early changes (0–3 months)
Gradual improvement in bone marrow edema is generally expected after VA. Although reduction in edema is greatest in the first 3 months after VA, most treated vertebrae (65%) still show some persistent bone marrow edema if imaged during this period. To make this situation somewhat more complex, it is not uncommon (10%) to see no significant change in the extent of bone marrow edema, or even occasional progression of edema during this period in comparison with pre-VA, with the patient's pain profile improving all the while.[17] This relatively rapid pain improvement with persistent edema could be explained by a lack of motion at the fracture site caused by fixation by cement while the fracture healing continues. When bone marrow edema is also seen within an adjacent vertebra on post-VA MR images, the differential diagnosis includes an acute adjacent-level vertebral fracture or infection.

Intermediate changes (3–6 months)
The resolution of bone marrow edema continues during this phase, but the rate slows down, with more than one-third (37%) of augmented vertebrae still showing some persistent edema.[17]

Late changes (6–12 months)
There is further gradual reduction in bone marrow edema during this period. Up to 29% of treated vertebrae can still show persistent edema. As seen in earlier stages, a decrease in the extent of bone marrow edema is not directly related to the improvement of back pain after VA.[17]

MR imaging and contrast enhancement Post-VA contrast enhancement changes on MR imaging, within and about treated vertebrae, shares many similarities with other features apparent after spine surgical procedures. Contrast enhancement occurs within the treated vertebra and may surround the injected cement. The enhancement pattern is fairly intense, especially on fat-suppressed T1-weighted sequences, but is variable in distribution and may extend along the needle tract(s). As is seen with bone marrow edema, contrast enhancement can be observed as a late change in post-VA imaging studies.

Bright rim sign As the bone marrow edema resolves, many treated vertebrae demonstrate a bright rim on STIR or T2-weighted images surrounding the cement cast. This bright rim becomes more apparent as the surrounding edema resolves, and can remain for several months. On T1-weighted

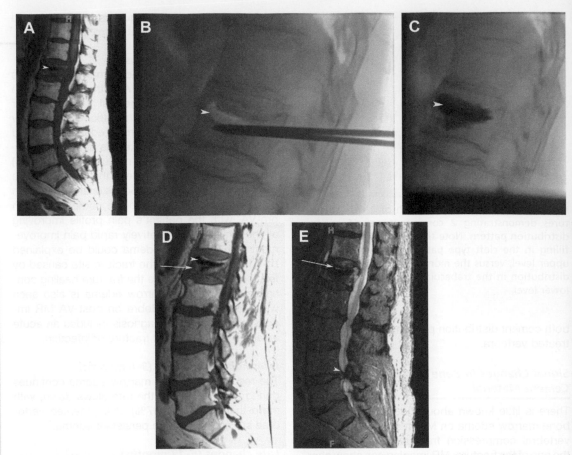

Fig. 7. An 84-year-old man presented with an acute L1 vertebral compression fracture with an inability to stand or walk. (*A*) Sagittal T1 image at the time of presentation shows diffuse edema with a cleft (*arrowhead*) in the upper part of the vertebral body. (*B*) Lateral fluoroscopic image during the VA procedure after the needle placement. Note that the cleft (*arrowhead*) appears bigger after the patient was positioned in hyperextension. (*C*) Post-VA image with expected cleft type cement-filling pattern (*arrowhead*). The patient had a dramatic improvement in the pain within a few hours and was able to stand and walk. (*D*) Two weeks later the patient presented with new low back pain, different in nature and lower in location than his previous pain. Two-week post-VA sagittal T1-weighted image shows the low signal intensity of the cement (*arrowhead*) within the vertebral body (*arrow*). Note that there is persistence of bone marrow edema while the pain from fracture was almost nonexistent. (*E*) Two-week post-VA short-tau inversion recovery (STIR) image shows bright rim sign with linear high signal intensity around the cement (*arrow*). His new pain was due to worsening of the disc herniation and central canal stenosis at the L4-L5 level (*arrowhead*).

images, the signal intensity of the rim is equal to that of water (early) or fat (later). The pathogenesis of this bright rim has been explained as a result of the exothermic reaction that happens during the

bone cement hardening within the vertebral body. As the temperature is highest in tissue directly in contact with the cement, this rim probably represents small necrotic areas surrounding the cement cast characterized by fatty infiltration of bone marrow.[21]

Another common imaging finding is linear high T2 and STIR signal in the path of the needle placement. This feature can also persist for several months, and generally improves gradually over time. It is likely of no clinical significance unless it is associated with fracture of the pedicle, and should not be confused with any new abnormality (**Fig. 8**).

Box 3
Categories of temporal changes in post-VA bone marrow edema on MR imaging

1. Early: 0 to 3 months post VA
2. Intermediate: 3 to 6 months post VA
3. Late: 6 to 12 months post VA

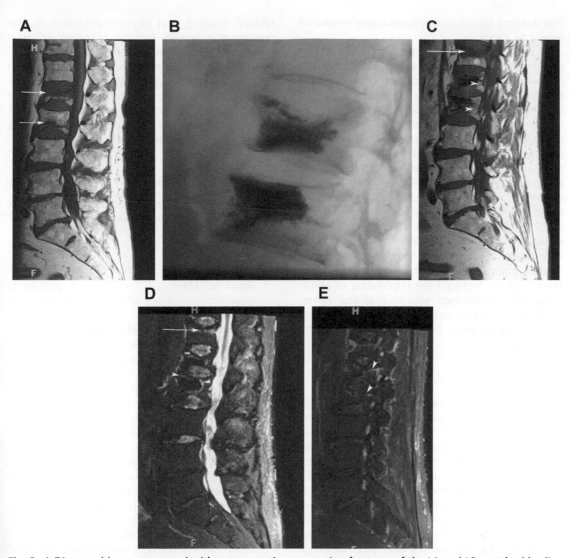

Fig. 8. A 71-year-old man presented with osteoporotic compression fractures of the L1 and L2 vertebral bodies. (*A*) Sagittal T1-weighted image shows fractures with edema (*arrows*). (*B*) Post-VA image shows cement distribution within the L1 and L2 vertebral bodies. The patient had significant improvement in pain but presented with recurrent back pain 3 weeks later. (*C*) Follow-up MR image shows new fracture at T12 (*arrow*) that explained his new symptoms. Note the significant improvement in edema surrounding the cement noticed in previously treated levels (*arrowheads*). (*D*) STIR image from 3-week post-VA follow-up MR demonstrates bright rim sign at the previous treatment level with well-demarcated hyperintense linear signal (*arrowheads*) surrounding the cement. Also seen is the new vertebral compression fracture at T12 (*arrow*). (*E*) STIR image from 3-week post-VA follow-up MR in para-midline position shows the linear hyperintense signal along the needle track at the treated levels.

Changes in Vertebral Size and Morphology

A VA procedure provides some immediate restoration of height and improvement of the wedge angle in the compressed vertebrae.[22] However, vertebral bodies can continue to lose some additional height after augmentation treatment. This further compression subsequent to treatment may or may not cause new symptoms.[15]

To date, no published prospective studies have examined this aspect. However, in a retrospective evaluation of 45 patients, 18% of successfully treated vertebral bodies had additional height loss of treated vertebrae without any recurrence of preprocedure symptoms. These patients presented with new symptoms that were different from their initial symptoms at the time of VA, and were explained by additional pathologic entities.

The average height loss in these cases measured from 1 to 2 mm.[15]

In a separate retrospective study, 6 of 250 patients who were treated with VA returned with renewed complaints of back pain after the initial improvement of symptoms for varying amounts of time.[23] The recurrent pain in these patients was similar to that experienced at the initial presentation before vertebroplasty. This renewed pain was attributed to new fractures within the previously treated vertebrae, possibly occurring around deposited cement. All patients were offered a repeat vertebroplasty based on the same workup as previously performed for the initial treatment, including medical history, physical examination, and appropriate imaging studies. After repeat treatment, 5 of the 6 patients demonstrated improvement in their recurrent pain.[23] These studies highlight the importance of correlating imaging findings with new clinical symptoms, physical examination, and other available relevant information to arrive at an accurate diagnosis.

EVALUATION OF NEW POST-VA PAIN

Presentation with renewed back pain after initial successful VA is common. Back pain is subjective, often multifactorial, and can be further complicated by a chronic course and associated comorbid conditions. Furthermore, it is often difficult for patients to precisely localize their back pain; hence, they attribute their back pain to a "failed" VA procedure. The knowledge of the expected imaging appearance "within the expected normal range" described in the previous section can be helpful in evaluating patients who return for imaging after VA with recurrent or residual pain of uncertain origin.

This new pain could result from a new compression fracture or several other abnormalities.[16] Plain radiography may or may not show a new vertebral compression fracture. Follow-up MR imaging should be strongly considered in patients with unexplained new or residual symptoms. MR imaging is not only helpful in identifying new compression fractures with bone marrow edema, but also other potential disorders such as facet arthritis, disc herniation, infection, and central canal stenosis.[15] Examination of patients and a thorough evaluation of their pain profiles and diagrams are also helpful. Fluoroscopic evaluation, when available, is also valuable, as it may be possible to readily identify a new vertebral compression deformity or a painful facet or sacroiliac joint.

The potential for a refracture of a vertebra after VA should be considered with appropriate clinical history, imaging, and physical examination. The presentation would include a recurrent pain consistent with the level of prior VA, and progression of height loss and marrow edema with no other explainable cause on MR imaging. Progressive and persistent edema and interval height loss after successful VA are common, and should not be interpreted as sufficient evidence of ongoing abnormality at the treated vertebral level.[15]

ACKNOWLEDGMENTS

Special thanks are extended to Dr Orlando Ortiz for providing some clinical examples.

REFERENCES

1. Riggs BL, Melton LJ. The worldwide problem of osteoporosis: insights afforded by epidemiology. Bone 1999;17:505S–11S.
2. Jensen ME, Evans AJ, Mathis JM, et al. Percutaneous polymethyl-methacrylate vertebroplasty in the treatment of osteoporotic vertebral body compression fractures: technical aspects. AJNR Am J Neuroradiol 1997;18:1897–904.
3. Mathis JM, Barr JD, Belkoff SM, et al. Percutaneous vertebroplasty: a developing standard of care for vertebral compression fractures. AJNR Am J Neuroradiol 2001;22:373–81.
4. Do HM. Magnetic resonance imaging in the evaluation of patients for percutaneous vertebroplasty. Top Magn Reson Imaging 2000;11:235–44.
5. Murphy KJ, Deramond H. Percutaneous vertebroplasty in benign and malignant disease. Neuroimaging Clin N Am 2000;10:535–45.
6. Mathis JM. Percutaneous vertebroplasty: complication avoidance and technique optimization. AJNR Am J Neuroradiol 2003;24:1697–706.
7. Cotton A, Dewatre F, Cortet B, et al. Percutaneous vertebroplasty for osteolytic metastasis and myeloma: effects of the percentage of lesion filling and the leakage of methyl methacrylate at clinical follow-up. Radiology 1996;200:525–30.
8. Cotton A, Boutry N, Cortet B, et al. Percutaneous vertebroplasty: state of the art. Radiographics 1998;18:311–20.
9. Padovani B, Kasriel O, Brunner P, et al. Pulmonary embolism caused by acrylic cement: a rare complication of percutaneous vertebroplasty. AJNR Am J Neuroradiol 1999;20:375–7.
10. Lin EP, Ekholm S, Hiwatashi A, et al. Vertebroplasty: cement leakage into the disc increases the risk of new fracture of adjacent vertebral body. AJNR Am J Neuroradiol 2004;25:175–80.
11. Nevitt MC, Ross PD, Palermo L, et al. Vertebral fractures, bone density and alendronate treatment with

incident vertebral fractures: effect of number and spinal location of fractures. Bone 1999;25:613–9.

12. Klazen CA, Venmans A, De Veries J, et al. Percutaneous vertebroplasty is not a risk factor for new osteoporotic compression fractures: results from VERTOS II. AJNR Am J Neuroradiol 2010;31:1447–50.

13. Papanastassiou ID, Phillips FM, Van Meirhaeghe J, et al. Comparing effects of kyphoplasty, vertebroplasty, and non-surgical management in a systematic review of randomized and non-randomized controlled studies. Eur Spine J 2012;21:1826–43.

14. Mathis JM, Percutaneous vertebroplasty: complication avoidance and tricks of the trade. AJNR Am J Neuroradiol 2002;24.119–20.

15. Dansie DM, Luetmer PH, Lane JI, et al. MRI findings after successful vertebroplasty. AJNR Am J Neuroradiol 2005;26:1595–600.

16. Kamalian S, Bordia R, Ortiz AO. Post-vertebral augmentation back pain: evaluation and management. AJNR Am J Neuroradiol 2012;33:370–5.

17. Voormolen MH, Van Rooij WJ, Van der Graaf Y, et al. Bone marrow edema in osteoporotic vertebral compression fractures after percutaneous vertebroplasty and relation with clinical outcome. AJNR Am J Neuroradiol 2006;27:983–8.

18. Fossaceaca R, Di Terlizzi M, Stecco A, et al. MRI post-vertebroplasty. Radiol Med 2007;112(2):185–94.

19. Tanigawa N, Komemushi A, Kariya S, et al. Relationship between cement distribution pattern and new compression fracture after percutaneous vertebroplasty. AJR Am J Roentgenol 2007;189:W348–52.

20. Baker LL, Goodman SB, Perkash I, et al. Benign versus pathologic compression fractures of vertebral bodies: assessment with conventional spin-echo, chemical-shift, and STIR MR imaging. Radiology 1996;199:541–9.

21. Deramond H, Wright NT, Belkoff SM. Temperature elevation caused by bone cement polymerization during vertebroplasty. Bone 1999;25(Suppl 2):17S–21S.

22. Hiwatashi A, Westesson PL, Yoshiura T, et al. Kyphoplasty and vertebroplasty produce the same degree of height restoration. AJNR Am J Neuroradiol 2009;30:669–73.

23. Gaughen JR, Jensen ME, Schweickert PA, et al. The therapeutic benefit of repeat percutaneous vertebroplasty at previously treated vertebral levels. AJNR Am J Neuroradiol 2002;23:1657–61.

Optimized Imaging of the Postoperative Spine

Anne Marie McLellan, DO*, Simon Daniel, MD,
Idoia Corcuera-Solano, MD, Vivek Joshi, MD,
Lawrence N. Tanenbaum, MD

KEYWORDS

- Spine • Spine hardware • Postoperative spine • Dual energy • MR imaging • CT

KEY POINTS

- Few tasks in imaging are more challenging than that of optimizing evaluations of the instrumented spine.
- Applying these fundamental principles to postoperative spine computed tomography and magnetic resonance examinations will mitigate the challenges associated with metal implants and significantly improve image quality and consistency.
- Newer and soon-to-be-available imaging enhancements should provide improved visualization of tissues and hardware as multispectral imaging sequences continue to develop.

INTRODUCTION

There are few imaging tasks more challenging to the radiologist than optimizing evaluations of the instrumented spine as there is significant artifact induced by implanted metal devices on both magnetic resonance (MR) imaging and computed tomography (CT). MR imaging artifacts are mainly caused by volume magnetic susceptibility mismatch between metal devices and tissue. In CT, the issues are beam hardening and streak (BHS) artifacts. The purpose of this article is to describe the critical techniques for MR and CT imaging of the postoperative spine, focusing on key technical factor adjustments; the value of innovations, such as dual energy CT (DECT); and new MR techniques, such as metal artifact reduction and chemical shift imaging.

CT

Fundamental Factors

CT is a quick and effective imaging tool for the evaluation of the spine in postoperative patients and is commonly obtained to demonstrate the position of surgical hardware with respect to the adjacent bone, nerves, spinal canal, and vessels. CT is best suited to assess for hardware complications, such as malpositioning, disruption, and mechanical loosening, as well as to demonstrate cortical and trabecular bone continuity at fusion sites.[1] In addition, in those patients with recurrent symptoms who have contraindications to MR imaging, CT provides the sole cross-sectional imaging option. Although CT is effective in evaluating the postoperative spine, there are challenges posed by BHS artifacts associated with metallic hardware. Metal-related attenuation of the x-ray beam manifests as dark and bright bands that reduce the integrity of visualization of the hardware as well as the surrounding bone and soft tissues.[2] The artifact depends on both fixed and modifiable variables. Fixed variables are related to the hardware itself and include metal composition (increased density, increased artifact) and geometry (increased thickness, increased beam attenuation). Modifiable variables are generally related to the CT acquisition parameters and

Department of Neuroradiology, Icahn School of Medicine at Mount Sinai, 1 Gustave Levy Place, New York, NY 10029, USA
* Corresponding author.
E-mail address: anne.mclellan@mountsinai.org

Neuroimag Clin N Am 24 (2014) 349–364
http://dx.doi.org/10.1016/j.nic.2014.01.005
1052-5149/14/$ – see front matter © 2014 Elsevier Inc. All rights reserved.

include x-ray kilovolt peak (kVp), x-ray tube current, pitch, and image reconstruction parameters (**Table 1**).[1]

KVP

One of the most important modifiable variables is the x-ray kilovolt value. Increasing the x-ray kVp decreases x-ray beam attenuation from metal, thereby reducing artifact. The radiation dose is directly affected by an increase in kVp from 120 to 140, producing an approximately 40% increase in the dose to patients. Appropriate reduction in tube current (milliamps per second) compensates for the increase, maintaining the radiation dose. In general, a 15% increase in kVp should be accommodated by a 50% decrease in mAs. Note that as low contrast detectability is inversely related to the kVp used, there is a small tradeoff in image sensitivity with increases in kVp.

ITERATIVE RECONSTRUCTION

The use of iterative reconstruction (IR) techniques, ubiquitous on modern scanners, reduces the dose required to obtain an appropriately low noise image. The ability of IR to recognize and then remove noise has a modest positive impact on the artifacts produced by metal hardware (**Fig. 1**). Newer model-based IR techniques have an even greater impact on artifact reduction (**Fig. 2**).

SLICE THICKNESS

The most important scanning parameter with respect to the degree of beam hardening artifact is the acquisition slice profile (**Fig. 3**). With a

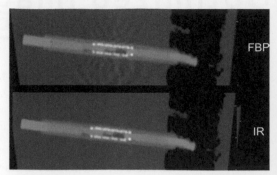

Fig. 1. Value of IR. Note the reduction of structured noise and artifact with the use of IR versus filtered back projection (FBP).

multichannel CT system, the minimum possible thickness should be fed to each imaging channel, as the benefit of the thinner acquisition voxels will be manifest in the in-plane, reformatted, and 3-dimensional (3D) images even if thicker slices are used for interpretive purposes. With increasing helical pitch (defined as table distance traveled per 360° rotation/total collimated width of the x-ray beam), slice profiles broaden; thus, minimum pitch values should be used. Techniques such as in-plane and through-plane oversampling lead to a reduction in effective voxel sizes and minimized artifact.

ADVANCED TECHNIQUES
DECT

Methods
Although the potential benefits have been known for some time, DECT has only recently become commercially available and practical over the last decade.[3] There are several commercially available methods for DECT,[4] including dual-source, single-source rapid voltage switching, single-source layered (also known as *sandwich*) detector, as well as sequential acquisition (spin-spin) (**Fig. 4**). Quantum counting detectors may be available in the future. Each method has advantages and disadvantages regarding spectral contrast and dose efficiency.[5]

Dual Source Imaging

Siemens Medical Corporation developed the first commercial dual-source approach based on 2 orthogonally mounted x-ray sources, which simultaneously expose a set of detectors (Somatom Definition Flash and Force). The second x-ray source is a smaller detector and, thus, has a relatively smaller field of view depending on the scanner model (see **Fig. 4**).[6]

Table 1	
Managing BHS artifact	
CT	**Managing Beam Hardening Artifact**
X-ray kVp	High kVp (110–120 kVp)
Image reconstruction algorithm	Model-based iterative reconstruction
Acquisition slice profile	Minimize voxel size High definition, oversampling
Dual energy	Dual source, single-source rapid voltage switching, single-source layered (sandwich) detector, sequential acquisition (spin-spin)

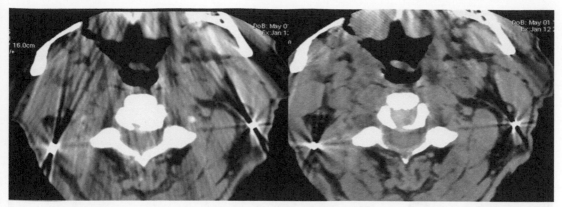

Fig. 2. Value of model-based IR: surgical clips and dental amalgam. Note the significant improvement of the spinal canal depiction with model-based IR (*right*) when compared with filtered back projection (*left*).

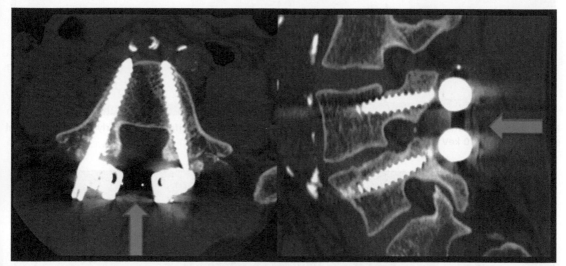

Fig. 3. Value of thin slices. Postoperative assessment on anterior decompression and fusion (16.0 × .625 mm). Note the low level of BHS associated with the spinal hardware with only minimal blooming and dark banding posteriorly (*arrow*).

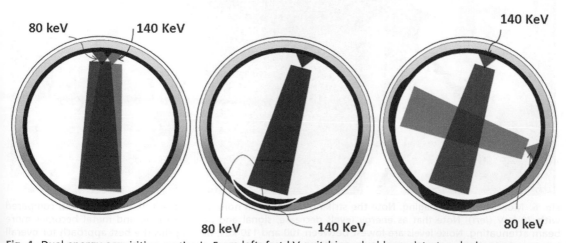

Fig. 4. Dual energy acquisition methods. From left: fast kV switching, dual layer detector, dual source.

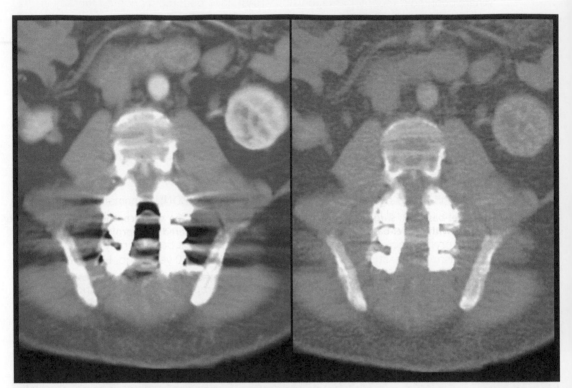

Fig. 5. Monochromatic imaging. Note the striking reduction in noise and artifact, particularly within the central spinal canal, at 110 keV (*right*) compared with 70 keV (*left*).

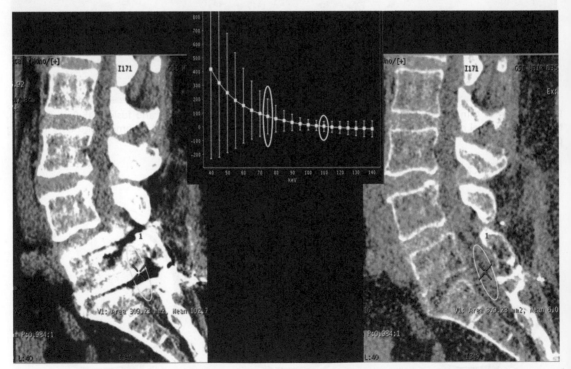

Fig. 6. Monochromatic imaging. Note the striking reduction in noise and artifact at 110 keV (*right*) compared with 70 keV (*left*). Note that as energy levels decrease, signal and noise increase, and metal becomes more beam attenuating. Noise levels are lowest between 100 and 110 keV, making this the best approach for overall imaging in the instrumented spine.

Fast Kilovolt Switching

General Electric Corporation introduced a different approach for acquiring DECT, termed *rapid voltage switching*. A single x-ray tube is used to generate alternating energy levels of 80 kVp and 140 kVp.[3] Energy switching at intervals of about 0.4 ms or less permits near simultaneous capture of both high-energy and low-energy CT information (see **Fig. 4**).

Dual-Layer Detector (Sandwiched Layers)

Phillips Corporation accomplishes DECT by using a detector specially designed to detect different energy levels in its dual sandwiched layers.[4] A single x-ray source is used at 120 to 140 keV. The superficial layer absorbs and detects most of the low-energy spectrum, which constitutes approximately 50% of the beam. The remaining high-energy photons penetrate to the deeper detector layer. Distinct CT images corresponding to the low and high energy levels are constructed from the single exposure (see **Fig. 4**).

Sequential Acquisition (Spin-Spin)

This approach involves conventional single-source hardware for the sequential acquisition of 2 data sets at low and then high kVp. A disadvantage is the delay between acquisitions presenting challenges with registration of respiratory, vascular, and cardiac motion as well as temporal variation in contrast opacification. This method is, thus, most viable for studies of the brain and spine and for delayed post–contrast agent infusion studies.[5]

Quantum Counting

Quantum counting detectors are capable of resolving the energies of individual impacting photons. The detectors use cadmium, zinc, telluride rather than the classic CT detector of tungsten.[7] These detectors are a focus of active investigation. At present their use has been restricted to small animal studies as they are not capable of the photon flux required for patient examinations and become quickly saturated.

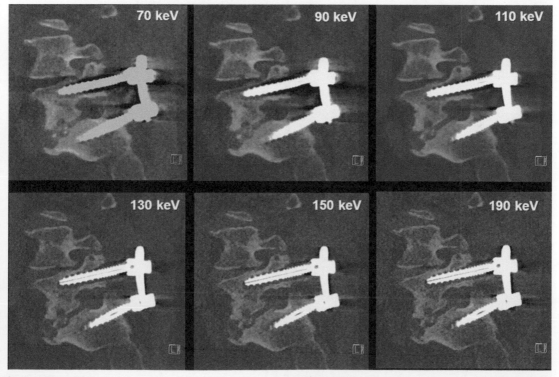

Fig. 7. Monoenergetic imaging: windowing by energy. Note that as the energy level increases, hardware visualization becomes more discrete with less blooming and better appreciation of the internal screw architecture. Low contrast detectability decreases at the highest energy levels while noise increases; thus, 110 keV is best for routine interrogation. The highest energy levels may add incremental information about the hardware itself and the immediately surrounding anchoring bone.

Output

Regardless of the method that is used, DECT energy involves obtaining image data at 2 distinct peak energy levels in contrast to the usual one.[2,8] Typical energy values used are 80 to 100 kVp for the lower and 140 to 150 kVp for the higher energy level, respectively.[9] By harvesting the tissue attenuation information at the extremes of energies, detailed material discrimination based on the atomic number can be extrapolated.

Diagnostic images based on individual materials (for example, iodine or hydroxyapatite) as well as at individual energies can be routinely reconstructed from these acquisitions. These monochromatic/monoenergetic data sets are selectable from 40 to 140/190 keV (depending on the scanner manufacturer) and vary significantly in appearance and character. In general, image sets obtained at mid energy levels (about 70 keV) provide a traditional appearance and low contrast detectability, whereas image sets obtained at

higher energy levels (about 110–190 keV) manifest reduced BHS artifact and, thus, improve the depiction of hardware (Fig. 5).[4]

Lower energy levels (about 40 keV) are more effectively attenuated by metals, such as iodine, less applicable in the instrumented spine but popular for contrast-enhanced examinations, such as CT angiography. Synthesized optimum contrast images combine the best features of the high- and low-energy beams into one diagnostic image.

The optimal monochromatic energy value will depend on whether one is interested in the best compromise energy to image all tissues or one is focused on imaging the implants and the anchoring osseous structures. A prior study suggests that 110 keV is the optimal compromise energy for the range of tissues in the spine, after instrumentation (Figs. 6 and 7).[10]

Preliminary research with General Electric's CT scanner's fast-kilovolt switching method suggests that monochromatic data sets in the energy

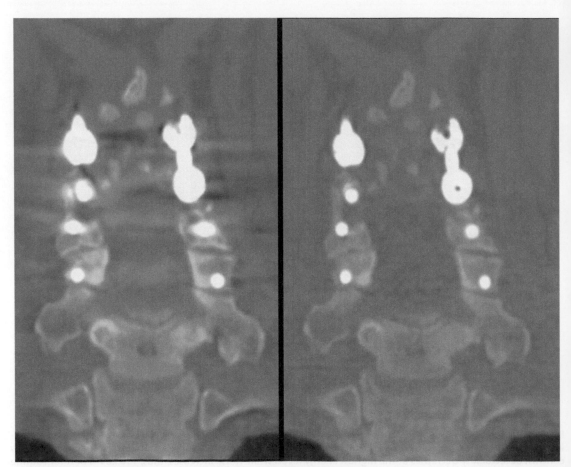

Fig. 8. Dual energy imaging of metal hardware. Note the more discrete and less distorted appearance of the hardware at 110 keV (*right*) compared with 70 keV (*left*).

range of 112 to 140 keV provide the best clarity of transpedicular screws and surrounding bony structures.[2] A different study using Siemens' dual-source CT found that the optimum energy values varied from 123 to 141 keV based on the location and composition of hardware (**Fig. 8**).[4]

As DECT methodologies differ between manufacturers, the precise optimal energy values/techniques for evaluating the postoperative spine and associated hardware may vary (**Figs. 9** and **10**).

MR IMAGING
Introduction

MR imaging lacks ionizing radiation and has superior soft tissue contrast resolution compared with CT. In addition, MR imaging is superior to CT in evaluating bone loss surrounding arthroplasties.[11] In the instrumented spine, MR imaging suffers from several challenges posed by regional anatomic distortion and failure of fat suppression (**Table 2**).

Managing Susceptibility

Metal artifacts result from the high magnetic susceptibility of hardware with respect to surrounding soft tissues. Materials used in biomedical implants include stainless steel, cobalt chrome, titanium, and rarely ultrahigh molecular weight polyethylene. Alloys that have less magnetic susceptibility are being trialed, including aluminum/platinum/niobium.[12] To best depict anchoring bone, surrounding soft tissues, and implanted hardware, one must minimize local susceptibility-based anatomic distortion and signal loss (see **Table 2**). Metallic implants disrupt the local static magnetic field (B), which then alters frequency-encoded and slice-selective image data. The local magnetic B_o perturbations produce images with a combination of signal loss, pixel pileup (seen as peripheral high signal) and distortion near metal implants leading to spatial mismapping of information.[13] The degree of distortion depends on the type of metal (for example, stainless steel is worse than titanium) as well as the field strength of the

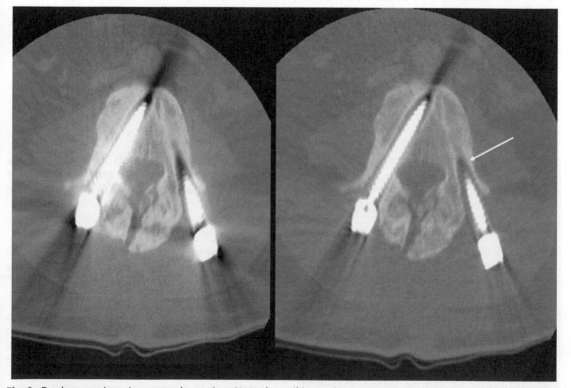

Fig. 9. Dual energy imaging: screw loosening. Note the striking reduction in BHS associated with the hardware at 110 keV (*right*) compared with 70 keV (*left*). The striking reduction of artifact greatly improves the depiction of the anchoring bone facilitating the diagnosis of loosening of the left-sided screw (*arrow*).

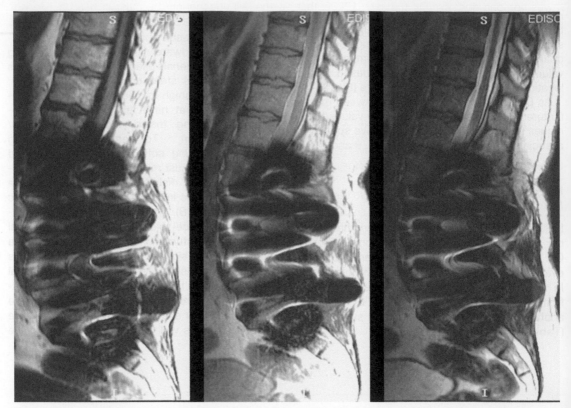

Fig. 10. High-susceptibility hardware. Note the severe distortion caused by this older metallic implant. Left to right: T1 spin echo (SE), proton density (PD) fast spin echo (FSE), T2 FSE at 1.5 T. Note the greater distortion on the T2 compared with the PD as artifact scales with echo time. Artifact is inversely related to echo train length; thus, the single echo short time to echo (TE) SE T1 shows more perturbation than do the longer TE fast/turbo spin echo images.

Table 2
Managing MR imaging susceptibility effects

MR	Managing Susceptibility
Bandwidth	Increase
Echo train length	Increase
Voxel size	Decrease
Frequency encoding direction	Adjust to A-P direction (parallel to long axis of pedicle screw)
Multispectral imaging	MAVRIC SEMAC/UTE

Abbreviations: A-P, anterior-to-posterior; FLAIR, fluid-attenuated inversion recovery; FSE, fast spin echo; MAVRIC, multi-acquisition with variable resonance image combination; SE, spin echo; SEMAC, slice-encoding metal artifact correction; UTE, ultrashort time to echo.

magnet. Susceptibility affects the scale, with the strength of the magnetic field producing particular challenges when scanning at 3 T (see **Fig. 10; Fig. 11**).[14]

MR Imaging Advanced Techniques

To optimize imaging of the instrumented spine, several fundamental principles should be considered.

Frequency Encoding Direction

Orientation of the frequency encoding direction along the long axis of the screw is generally the best tactic to minimize artifact. Typically this means frequency encoding in the anterior-to-posterior (A-P) direction on sagittal spine images. A-P frequency encoding may be the best solution for images in the axial plane as well (**Figs. 12–14**).[15]

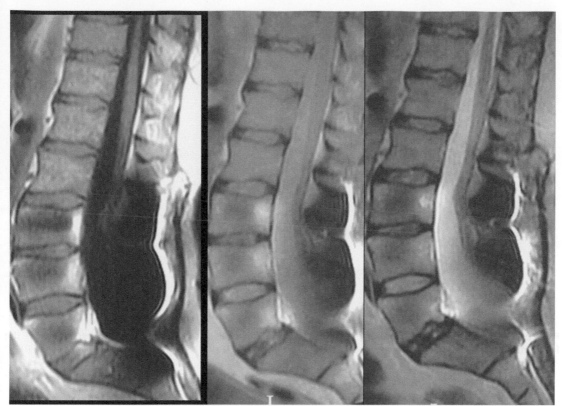

Fig. 11. High-susceptibility hardware. Left to right: T1 SE, PD FSE, T2 FSE at 0.2 T. Distortion related to susceptibility scales with field strength. Note the markedly reduced distortion caused by this older metallic implant. Artifact is inversely related to echo train length; thus, the single echo short TE SE T1 shows more perturbation than do the longer TE fast/turbo spin echo images.

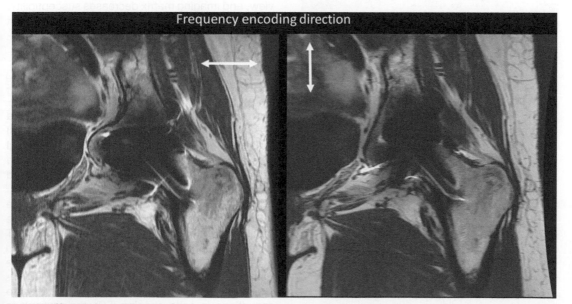

Fig. 12. Effect of frequency encoding orientation. Note the lateral distortion of screws and resurfaced head with right to left (R-L) encoding (*left*). Superior to inferior (S-I) encoding reduces the distortion from the screws and head.

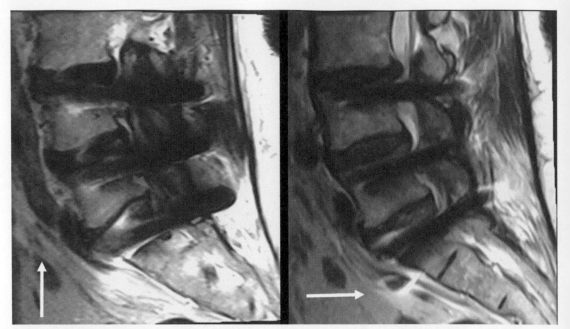

Fig. 13. Effect of frequency encoding direction. Note the more discrete appearance of the screws with the frequency encoding A-P (*right*) compared with superior inferior (SI) (*left*).

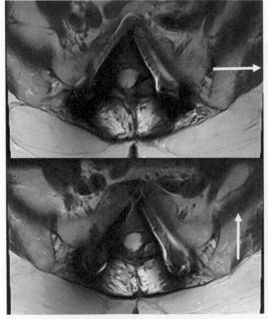

Fig. 14. Effect of frequency encoding direction. Note the more discrete appearance of the screws with the frequency encoding A-P (*bottom*) compared with right to left (RL) (*top*).

Small Voxel Sizes

Minimizing voxel size via slice thickness, field of view, and imaging matrix decreases susceptibility. The smallest voxel sizes are more practical at higher magnetic field strengths, partially ameliorating the potential for greater artifact (**Fig. 15**).[16]

High Bandwidth

Raising receiver bandwidth (BW) reduces susceptibility artifact. A doubling of the BW will lead to a 40% reduction in the signal-to-noise ratio (SNR) for a simple non–echo train acquisition. The signal loss can be compensated for with an increased number of scan averages at the cost of increased scan time. High BW scanning is common in modern spine protocols using high-density surface coils. This point is especially true at 3 T where the susceptibility effect is double that of 1.5 T and there is abundant signal to trade (**Fig. 16**).

Fortunately, several positive effects are associated with increases in BW, mitigating the theoretical loss in efficiency. As increases in BW lead to reductions in echo spacing (ES), the signal loss caused by T2 decay (proportional to ES × echo train length [ETL]) is substantially ameliorated.

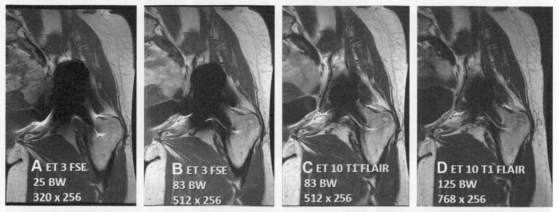

Fig. 15. Effect of bandwidth (BW), echo train length, and voxel size. Original acquisition at left (A). Note substantial reduction in distortion with large increase in BW and modest reduction in voxel size (B). Shift from echo train (ET) 3 to 10 leads to a marked improvement in image quality (C). An additional 50% increase in BW and modest decrease in voxel size further refines the image (D).

Higher BW levels improve slice readout efficiency, allowing lower time to repetition (TR) values per required number of slices and reducing the time penalty in averaging. The amount of blur perceptible on an echo train (ET) scan such as fast spin echo (FSE) is also proportional to ES × ETL. The shorter ES at higher BW is more suitable to longer ETLs, which independently reduce artifact (see later discussion). The use of longer ETLs can directly reduce the time per slice or allow the use of longer TR values at equal scan times. Longer TR values can improve SNR as there is more relaxation time for signal to recover also reducing the need for more scan averaging.[17]

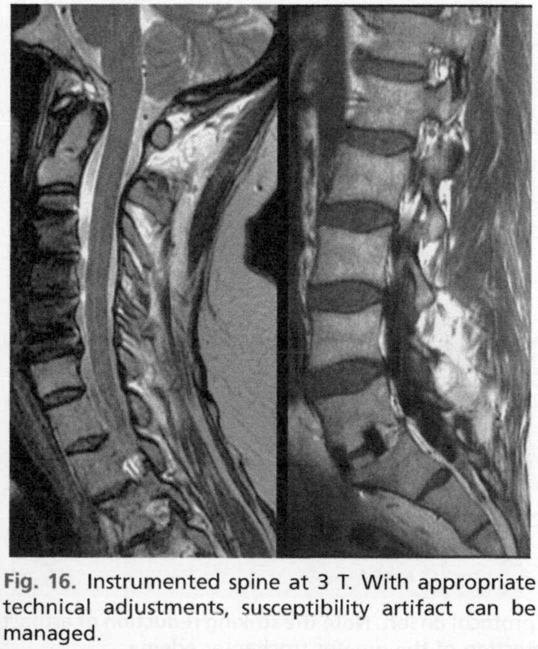

Fast/Turbo Spin Echo

Fast or turbo spin echo (F/TSE) sequences with echo trains are less susceptible to metal artifact than are the single-spin echo sequences. With F/TSE, each pulse (typically 180°) in an echo train has a refocusing effect on the tissue signal reducing signal loss and distortion. As F/TSE has been widely adopted for T2-weighted imaging, this advice has the greatest incremental benefit with T1-weighted acquisitions, which are commonly acquired with spin echo techniques. The alternate use of short ET FSE and longer ET T1 fluid-attenuated inversion recovery will significantly reduce the distorting effect of metal (see **Figs. 11** and **15**).

Issues at 3 T

Challenges at 3 T include proportionately greater susceptibility artifact along with doubled chemical shift effects. Very high BW levels (at least double of that used at 1.5 T) permit the use of longer ETL and reduces the chemical shift to that of a 1.5-T scanner. Higher SNR permits the routine use of smaller voxels. Leveraging the potentially doubled signal of 3 T will leave susceptibility effects similar to what can be seen at 1.5 T (see **Fig. 16**).

Fig. 16. Instrumented spine at 3 T. With appropriate technical adjustments, susceptibility artifact can be managed.

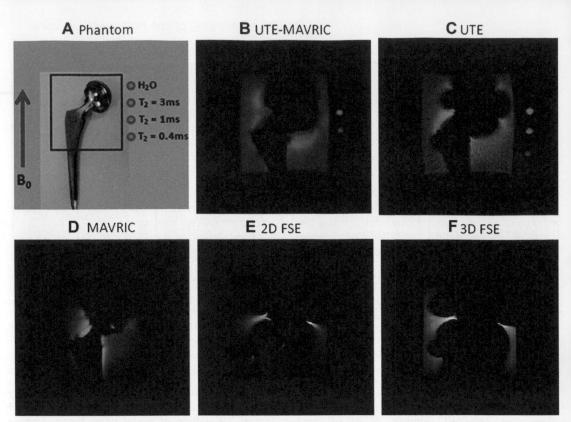

Fig. 17. Value of MSI and ultrashort time to echo (UTE). (*A*) Phantom images sequentially in (*B-F*). (*B*) UTE-Mavric sequence hybrid. (*C*) UTE. (*D*) Mavric alone. (*E*) 2D FSE (fast spin echo) 3D FSE. Note that (*B*) the hybrid sequence is optimal. (*From* Carl M, Koch K, Du J. MR imaging near metal with undersampled 3D radial UTE-MAVRIC sequences. Magn Reson Med 2013;69(1):27–36; with permission.)

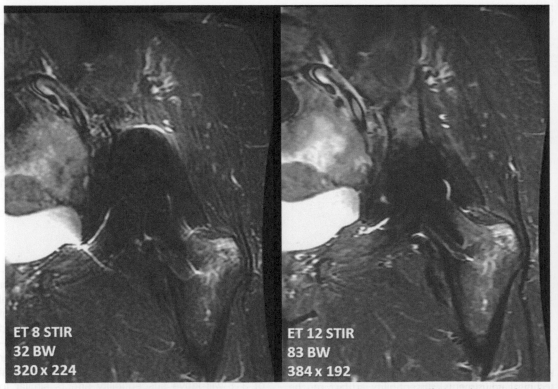

Fig. 18. Effect of parameter changes (BW and ET). Original protocol on left. Note the striking reduction of artifact and preservation of fat suppression with STIR allowing detection of the greater trochanter edema.

MULTISPECTRAL IMAGING

Novel imaging methods, such as multispectral or multi-sequence imaging (MSI), have been commercialized as MAVRIC (multi-acquisition with variable resonance image combination; GE Healthcare, Little Chalfont, United Kingdom) and SEMAC (slice-encoding metal artifact correction; Siemens Medical Corporation). These 3D sequences directly correct distortion effects over a range of offset frequencies near metal by employing using an alternative spectral and 3D spatial-encoding scheme whereby the signal is divided into bins and then controlled.[18,19] These techniques are effective in visualizing anatomy that would be obscured with conventional imaging, but the overall scan times tend be longer.[20]

ULTRASHORT TIME TO ECHO

A pitfall of routine sequences based on FSE is the suboptimal detection of tissues with very short T2 characteristics. Ultrashort time to echo (UTE) imaging techniques are capable of dramatic depiction of structures, such as tendons, ligaments, and cortical bone, and can be used as part of an MSI acquisition offering combined benefits.[21] As distortion is related to echo time, UTE leads to a dramatic reduction in artifact (Fig. 17).

Fat Suppression

As fat suppression is commonly used to augment contrast-enhanced imaging and is essential for the preservation of contrast resolution on T2-weighted studies of bone and extracanalicular soft tissues, one must manage metal-associated, regional susceptibility-based failures. Commonly used radiofrequency (RF)-based fat suppression techniques are highly prone to failure in the presence of the field-disturbing effects of metal. Similarly, when body shape varies significantly, such as at the cervicothoracic junction, RF fat suppression tends to fail.

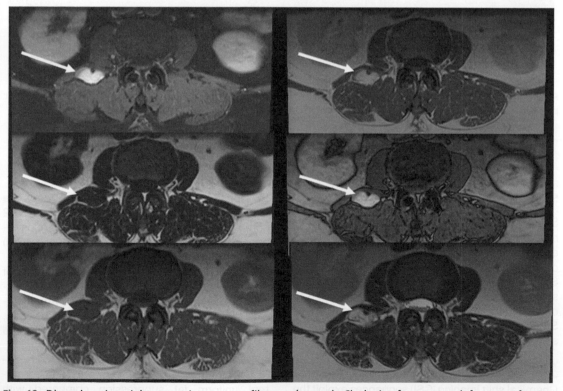

Fig. 19. Dixon imaging right paraspinous neurofibroma (*arrows*). Clockwise from upper left: water-fat suppressed, in phase, out of phase, T2-weighted, T1-weighted spin echo, fat only. Note the additional value of the in-phase image, which facilitates comparison with the non–fat-suppressed precontrast scan. Fat suppression shifts the image dynamic range and can lead to overestimation of enhancement.

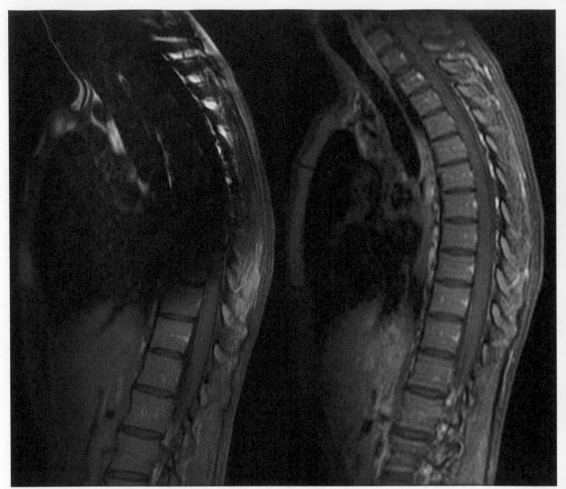

Fig. 20. CSI and fat suppression. Note the regional failure in fat suppression with RF techniques in this pediatric patient. The IDEAL water-only image (*right*) provides uniform suppression.

STIR

Short tau inversion (STIR) techniques are highly resistant to these regional fat-suppression failures and offer robust combined T2- and T1-weighted contrast ideal for imaging bone disease. Because STIR suppresses the signal of all tissue with a short T1 time, the technique is not applicable to contrast-enhanced studies. STIR studies can be SNR challenged unless scan times are lengthy or spatial resolution is reduced (**Fig. 18**).

Chemical Shift Fat Suppression

Chemical shift imaging (CSI) sequences exploit the differences in precession velocities of fat and water protons.[22] Fat and water proton signals vary according to resonant frequency or chemical shift.

By isolating these components into 2 separate images and then adding and subtracting the 2 complex images from in-phase and opposed-phase imaging, selective water (fat suppressed) and fat images can be created (**Fig. 19**).

Techniques such as iterative decomposition of water and fat with echo asymmetry and least-squares estimation (IDEAL) and DIXON are chemical shift methods that, among other benefits, provide robust fat suppression for both T1- and T2-weighted studies (**Fig. 20**).

CSI acquisitions are insensitive to the inhomogeneity of the magnetic field, thus providing consistent uniform fat suppression compared with conventional fat-saturation methods (**Fig. 21**).[23] The disadvantage is increased acquisition time, particularly for 3-point methods as 3 sequential

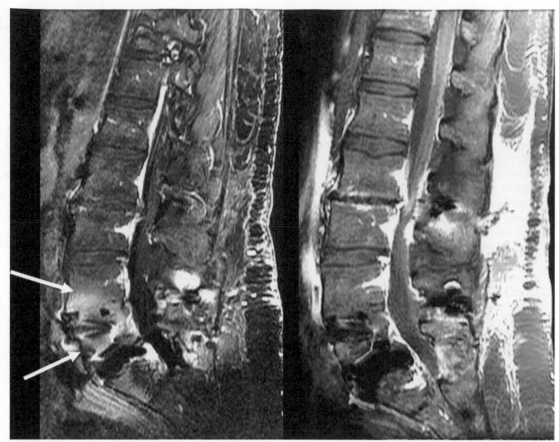

Fig. 21. CSI and fat suppression. RF fat suppression (*left*) shows localized failures about the L4-5 spacer (*arrows*) creating the impression of enhancement in the adjacent vertebral bodies. IDEAL water-only study shows more uniform suppression of fat signal and avoids the pseudoenhanced appearance. Note the accidental swapping of the frequency encoding direction to superior to interior on the right, which creates a larger appearance of the metallic implants at the L4-S1 disk spaces and posteriorly.

acquisitions are necessary. Techniques such as parallel imaging and high BW scanning have reduced much of the time penalty.[24]

SUMMARY

Few tasks in imaging are more challenging than that of optimizing evaluations of the instrumented spine. Applying these fundamental principles to postoperative spine CT and MR examinations will mitigate the challenges associated with metal implants and significantly improve image quality and consistency. Newer and soon-to-be-available imaging enhancements should provide improved visualization of tissues and hardware as MSI sequences continue to develop.

REFERENCES

1. Stradiotti P, Curti A, Castellazzi G, et al. Metal-related artifacts in instrumented spine. Techniques for reducing artifacts in CT and MRI: state of the art. Eur Spine J 2009;18(Suppl 1):102–8.
2. Srinivasan A, Hoeffner E, Ibrahim M, et al. Utility of dual-energy CT virtual keV monochromatic series for the assessment of spinal transpedicular hardware-bone interface. AJR Am J Roentgenol 2013;201(4):878–83.
3. Johnson TR. Dual energy CT in clinical practice. Berlin: Springer-Verlag; 2011.
4. Krasnicki T, Podgorski P, Guzinski M, et al. Novel clinical applications of dual energy computed tomography. Adv Clin Exp Med 2012;21(6):831–41.
5. Johnson TR. Dual-energy CT: general principles. AJR Am J Roentgenol 2012;199(Suppl 5):S3–8.
6. Karcaaltincaba M, Aktas A. Dual-energy CT revisited with multidetector CT: review of principles and clinical applications. Diagn Interv Radiol 2011;17(3):181–94.
7. Le Huy Q, Ducote JL, Molloi S. Radiation dose reduction using a CdZnTe-based computed

tomography system: comparison to flat-panel detectors. Med Phys 2010;37(3):1225–36.

8. White LM, Buckwalter KA. Technical considerations: CT and MR imaging in the postoperative orthopedic patient. Semin Musculoskelet Radiol 2002;6(1):5–17.

9. Guggenberger R, Winklhofer S, Osterhoff G, et al. Metallic artefact reduction with monoenergetic dual-energy CT: systematic ex vivo evaluation of posterior spinal fusion implants from various vendors and different spine levels. Eur Radiol 2012; 22(11):2357–64.

10. Tanenbaum L. Dual energy spectral CT of the instrumented spine: tuned monochromatic imaging improves quality over traditional techniques. American Society of Neuroradiology annual meeting. Seattle, June 4–9, 2011.

11. Awh M. Hip athroplasty. MRI web clinic. 2011. Available at: http://www.radsource.us/clinic/1102. Accessed October 31, 2013.

12. Uyama E, Inui S, Hamada K, et al. Magnetic susceptibility and hardness of Au-xPt-yNb alloys for biomedical applications. Acta Biomater 2013;9(9): 8449–53.

13. Koff MF, Shah P, Koch KM, et al. Quantifying image distortion of orthopedic materials in magnetic resonance imaging. J Magn Reson Imaging 2013; 38(3):610–8.

14. Graf H, Lauer UA, Berger A, et al. RF artifacts caused by metallic implants or instruments which get more prominent at 3 T: an in vitro study. Magn Reson Imaging 2005;23(3):493–9.

15. Hargreaves BA, Worters PW, Pauly KB, et al. Metal-induced artifacts in MRI. AJR Am J Roentgenol 2011;197(3):547–55.

16. Guermazi A, Miaux Y, Zaim S, et al. Metallic artefacts in MR imaging: effects of main field orientation and strength. Clin Radiol 2003;58(4):322–8.

17. Chen CA, Chen W, Goodman SB, et al. New MR imaging methods for metallic implants in the knee: artifact correction and clinical impact. J Magn Reson Imaging 2011;33(5):1121–7.

18. Hayter CL, Koff MF, Shah P, et al. MRI after arthroplasty: comparison of MAVRIC and conventional fast spin-echo techniques. AJR Am J Roentgenol 2011;197(3):W405–11.

19. Bydder GM, Pennock JM, Steiner RE, et al. The short TI inversion recovery sequence–an approach to MR imaging of the abdomen. Magn Reson Imaging 1985;3(3):251–4.

20. Lu W, Pauly KB, Gold GE, et al. SEMAC: slice encoding for metal artifact correction in MRI. Magn Reson Med 2009;62(1):66–76.

21. Carl M, Koch K, Du J. MR imaging near metal with undersampled 3D radial UTE-MAVRIC sequences. Magn Reson Med 2013;69(1):27–36.

22. Cha JG, Hong HS, Park JS, et al. Practical application of iterative decomposition of water and fat with echo asymmetry and least-squares estimation (IDEAL) imaging in minimizing metallic artifacts. Korean J Radiol 2012;13(3):332–41.

23. Costa DN, Pedrosa I, McKenzie C, et al. Body MRI using IDEAL. AJR Am J Roentgenol 2008;190(4): 1076–84.

24. Reeder SB, Pineda AR, Wen Z, et al. Iterative decomposition of water and fat with echo asymmetry and least-squares estimation (IDEAL): application with fast spin-echo imaging. Magn Reson Med 2005;54(3):636–44.

Imaging and Management of Postoperative Spine Infection

Joseph P. Mazzie, DO[a],*, Michael K. Brooks, MD, MPH[b],
Jeffrey Gnerre, MD[c]

KEYWORDS

- Postoperative spine • Infection • Spondylodiskitis • Epidural abscess • Spine surgery

KEY POINTS

- Evaluation of postoperative spine infection is a challenging task that requires a systematic approach for the accurate interpretation of spine imaging studies.
- Distinguishing between postsurgical inflammatory changes and spondylodiskitis, as well as infected postoperative fluid collections, is crucial for successful interpretation and successful patient management.

INTRODUCTION

Evaluation of potential complications in the postoperative spine is a challenging assignment and is the responsibility of many radiologists on a daily basis. The growth in surgical spine intervention has driven the advancement and use of multimodality imaging of the preoperative and postoperative spine. The radiologist interpreting postoperative spine examinations is presented with difficult conditions related to metallic instrumentation and implants, which result in artifacts obscuring anatomic detail, as well as the difficulties in distinguishing postsurgical inflammation from infection.[1,2] Despite preprocedure antibiotic prophylaxis and improved surgical techniques and postoperative care, as well as advances in multimodality diagnostic imaging, postoperative infectious complications result in significant morbidity and occasional mortality.[3] The diagnosis and management of postoperative spine infections are dependent on the assessment of multimodality imaging.

Postoperative spine infections are classified as either superficial or deep. Infectious processes contained within the skin and subcutaneous tissues without fascial involvement such as cellulitis or subcutaneous abscess are considered superficial. Deep infections occur deep to the lumbodorsal fascia for posterior lumbar wounds and deep to the ligamentum nuchae for posterior cervical wounds. Spondylodiskitis, epidural abscess, and paravertebral collections with superimposed infections are considered deep infections.[4,5]

RADIOGRAPHY

Baseline postoperative radiographs show initial implant positioning and may be used for future comparison in patients suspected of developing complications. Although plain radiography is insensitive in the detection of early postoperative infection, it still remains the initial imaging modality for postoperative evaluation, because fusion status, spinal stability, or hardware failure can all be shown on serial radiographs.[6] The limited usefulness of plain radiography is because of a lack of sensitivity to the early findings of infection within both the soft tissues of the spine and the spine proper. Fluoroscopy does serve as a useful modality in performing image-guided percutaneous biopsy of the spinal axis, particularly in the lumbar spine.

[a] Department of Radiology, Winthrop-University Hospital, 259 First Street, Mineola, NY 11501, USA; [b] Division of Musculoskeletal and Interventional Radiology, Stony Brook University School of Medicine, Stony Brook, NY 11794, USA; [c] New York Medical College at Westchester Medical Center, Valhalla, NY 10595, USA
* Corresponding author.
E-mail address: jmazzie@winthrop.org

Neuroimag Clin N Am 24 (2014) 365–374
http://dx.doi.org/10.1016/j.nic.2014.01.003
1052-5149/14/$ – see front matter © 2014 Elsevier Inc. All rights reserved.

COMPUTED TOMOGRAPHY

Most spine procedures use metallic instrumentation, with the goal of providing stability and reducing pain. Multidetector computed tomography (MDCT) is an excellent modality for assessing orthopedic spinal hardware complications.[7] In the early postoperative period, MDCT can effectively evaluate spinal alignment and implant positioning in relation to adjacent cortical bone, thecal sac, and neural foramina.[8] In the late postoperative period, MDCT can evaluate the progression of osseous fusion and bone graft incorporation. However, computed tomography (CT), like radiography, cannot readily distinguish the early findings of infection from the typical soft tissue, disk, and osseous changes that are encountered after spine surgery. With time, as is also seen in radiography, increased soft tissue swelling or induration, abnormal fluid collections, and osseous destruction may be seen on CT. Yet, the diagnosis of spine infection is usually established at this point in the patient's clinical course. CT does serve as a useful modality to guide spine biopsy throughout the spinal axis in cases of suspected spine infection.

ULTRASONOGRAPHY

Sonography has a limited role in postoperative infection imaging with its primary usefulness in detection of postoperative fluid collections and abscesses. In addition, sonography could be used for imaging guidance aspirations of these superficial fluid collections when the diagnosis of infection of a collection needs to be excluded.[6]

MAGNETIC RESONANCE IMAGING

Magnetic resonance (MR) imaging has an increasing role in imaging postoperative patients with suspected infection, both without and with spinal hardware. Advances in MR imaging technology and pulse sequence development have facilitated imaging in postoperative patients because of its superior soft tissue resolution.[9,10] Assessment of bone marrow edema, soft tissue signal changes and enhancement, and identification of abnormal fluid collections are more accurately and consistently detected with MR imaging than with other imaging modalities.[9] MR imaging is particularly useful for detecting and monitoring osteomyelitis/diskitis and postoperative fluid collections.[10] Typically, imaging of implants/spinal hardware produces geometric distortion, the so-called susceptibility artifact, which is caused by the differences in the magnetic properties of human tissue and those of the implanted hardware.[11] Titanium implants, which have been increasingly used, are nonferromagnetic and produce fewer artifacts than those made of ferromagnetic materials, such as stainless steel. Nonmetallic devices, such as nonmetallic interbody spacers, produce little artifact on MR imaging.[10] However, visualization of infectious disease that is close to hardware remains a challenge.[11] One technique that can be used to reduce artifact from implants is to align the main magnetic field (z-axis of the scanner) parallel with the long axis of the implanted hardware. Typically, this technique is more easily used in open magnets, where there is less restriction on patient positioning within the bore.[11] Several other techniques are available and have proved to reduce hardware artifact, including increasing the frequency encoding gradient strength, decreasing voxel size, increasing bandwidth, and decreasing field strength.

NUCLEAR MEDICINE

Nuclear medicine studies can also be used as part of the diagnostic workup of suspected spinal infection. These studies include 3-phase bone scans, gallium scans, and indium-111 leukocyte studies. These examinations are typically used in select situations, despite their high sensitivity and specificity, largely secondary to their poor spatial resolution and lengthy duration of the examinations. The current radionuclide imaging method of choice for diagnosing spinal osteomyelitis is combined bone-gallium imaging studies, which have been shown to be comparable with MR imaging.[12] Uptake that is greater or discordant on gallium imaging compared with technetium (bone scan) is the most accurate finding for spondylodiskitis. Typically, this examination combination (bone-gallium scan) is used in patients in whom MR imaging is contraindicated or in whom MR imaging and CT are equivocal (Fig. 1). Gallium single-photon emission CT can be comparable with combined bone-gallium imaging for diagnosing osteomyelitis.[13] Fluorodeoxyglucose positron emission tomography also seems to be useful in diagnosing spinal osteomyelitis, with high sensitivities and specificities, although the data sample size is small.[14]

SPONDYLODISKITIS/EPIDURAL ABSCESS

Spondylodiskitis is a term that encompasses a spectrum of infectious processes within the spine, including vertebral osteomyelitis and diskitis. Spinal column infections occur via several different routes, with direct hematogenous seeding of the vertebral bodies being the most common pathway. In adults, end arterioles are the vascular supply to the vertebral body subchondral

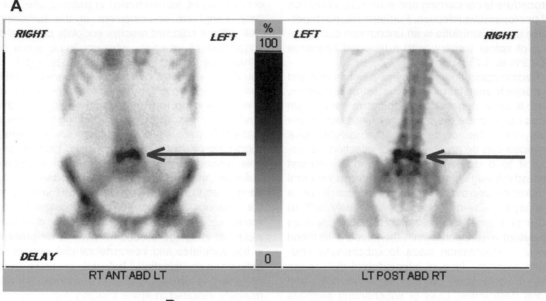

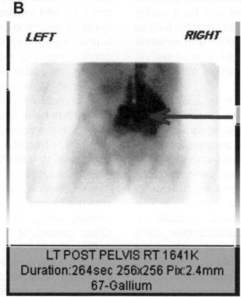

Fig. 1. Spondylodiskitis. (*A*) Bone scan and (*B*) gallium scans. Images from the delayed portion of a 3-phase bone scan show increased uptake at L5-S1 (*arrow*), with corresponding activity on the gallium scan images (*arrow*).

endplates, with the adjacent intervertebral disks receiving nutrients via simple diffusion. Therefore, hematogenous seeding of vertebral body infection occurs at the level of the end arterioles adjacent to the subchondral endplates, with pyogenic infection subsequently spreading from the endplate into the adjacent intervertebral disk. Hematogenous spread may also occur via epidural venous extension. Direct inoculation stemming from penetrating trauma or direct exposure from open wounds, previous spinal surgery, and diagnostic and therapeutic interventional procedures, as well as contiguous spread from adjacent soft

tissue infection, are other known routes of spinal column inoculation.[15,16] Untreated infection can spread into adjacent soft tissues, resulting in paravertebral, psoas, and epidural abscess formation.

The diagnosis of postoperative spine infection is based on clinical, laboratory, and radiologic features. Complaints of vague or increasing neck or low back pain may be the only early indication of postprocedural diskitis. However, this complaint profile overlaps significantly with postoperative spine pain. Fever is an inconsistent sign of diskitis; however, a persistently increased C-reactive protein level for more than 2 weeks after a spine procedure is concerning and is an early indication of postoperative infection. Furthermore, postoperative spondylodiskitis is an uncommon complication of spinal surgery, with a reported incidence of 0.2% to 2.75%.[5]

Radiographic findings may take between 2 and 4 weeks to manifest after the onset of symptoms, and thus a negative postoperative radiograph does not exclude the presence of infection. However, in cases of postoperative diskitis, disk collapse can be an early sign of infection, occurring 4 to 6 weeks after surgery.[17] As infection spreads through and replaces the normal vertebral medullary marrow, a relative decrease in bone density may be detected. Approximately 30% to 40% of normal mineralization is usually needed to detect osteopenia within the infected vertebral body.[18] Progression leads to subchondral endplate erosions, loss of intervertebral disk space height, osteolysis surrounding hardware, and bone destruction. Loss of subchondral endplate definition or endplate erosions can be a subtle finding but is the most reliable radiographic feature in detecting underlying early diskitis with vertebral osteomyelitis.[18] Endplate sclerosis may be seen in the later stages of chronic infection, followed by fusion of the disk space.

Detection of endplate erosions and cortical discontinuity may be identified earlier with CT compared with plain films, as well as paraspinal inflammatory changes and psoas abscess formation with the addition of contrast-enhanced scans.[8,18] The latter study is not commonly performed, but is often considered when patients are not candidates for an MR imaging examination.

MR imaging remains the preferred modality for the evaluation of potential postoperative spine infections, in particular diskitis and epidural abscess. Nevertheless, differentiating postsurgical changes versus developing infection is challenging. Subchondral endplate irregularity and erosions may be seen as loss of the normal cortical bone on T1-weighted images. Bone marrow infiltration along the vertebral endplates is classically shown by hypointense T1 and hyperintense T2 signal, as well as enhancement on postcontrast images. Progression of infection through the endplates results in diskitis. Subsequent edema and purulent material in the disk space show hypointense T1 and hyperintense T2 signal (Fig. 2).[15] There is significant overlap of imaging findings between the postoperative spine and the infected postoperative spine. For example, after diskectomy, hyperintense T2 signal is seen within the intervertebral disk space and adjacent subchondral endplates. Varying amounts of intradiskal enhancement are seen after intravenous gadolinium

contrast agent administration in patients after surgery. Peripheral enhancement of the remaining disk without adjacent reactive endplate changes is suggestive of infection, whereas linear areas of enhancement are more likely postsurgical in cause.[9,19] Vertebral body and intervertebral disk space enhancement may normally be seen at 6 weeks and up to 6 months after surgery in the absence of infection.[20] An enhancing soft tissue mass in the paravertebral or epidural space is highly suggestive of septic spondylodiskitis.[21] Given variable appearances of disk enhancement and postoperative marrow changes, spondylodiskitis may be difficult to reliably diagnose on MR imaging in the absence of epidural or paravertebral abscesses.[22] Restricted diffusion using diffusion-weighted imaging has been shown to be present in the endplates and intervertebral disk spaces of patients with infection, but not in those with degenerative disease. Diffusion sequences are not routinely included in spine imaging protocols, but can be useful in cases in which there is a specific question regarding degeneration versus infection.[23]

Image-guided spine biopsy is often requested to confirm cases of suspected spondylodiskitis, as well as potentially isolating an organism to more specifically tailor antibiotic therapy. The accuracy rate for percutaneous image-guided disk space biopsy has been reported to be as low as 47.5% to 57% in the setting of surgically proven spondylodiskitis.[24] Negative biopsy results, defined as not being able to identify a causative microorganism, may be caused by several factors (Box 1). The most common cause of a negative biopsy is that the biopsy is performed when the patient is already being treated with antibiotic therapy. Other causes of a negative biopsy include insufficient specimen, improper specimen handling and processing, disk aspiration without obtaining subchondral bone, or a specimen sampled from a region not containing viable organisms. In adults, pyogenic spondylodiskitis originates at the level of vertebral endplates, with subsequent spread into adjacent intervertebral disks; thus, subchondral bone should be sampled during image-guided disk biopsy.[24] Positive identification of an organism after percutaneous disk biopsy allows for effective intravenous antibiotic treatment alone without surgical intervention.[5]

A critical step in the performance of image-guided spine biopsy in postoperative spine patients with suspected infection is to perform the procedure on an urgent basis, before the administration of antibiotic therapy. This strategy requires active communication between the radiologist, the surgeon, the internist, the infectious disease specialist, and the patient. All imaging studies

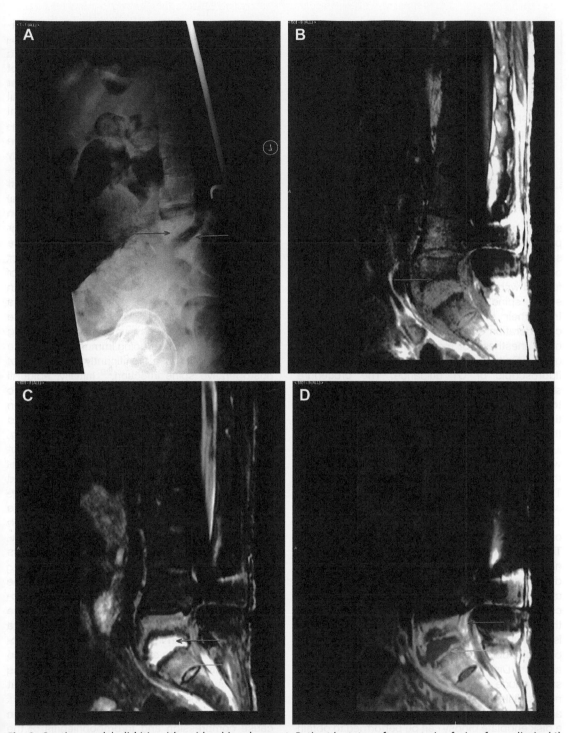

Fig. 2. Septic spondylodiskitis with epidural involvement. Patient is status after posterior fusion for scoliosis. (A) Lateral radiograph shows indistinctness of adjacent endplates, with considerable endplate sclerosis (*red arrows*). (B) Sagittal T1-weighted image shows obliteration of the disk space, with irregularity of contiguous endplates and loss of the cortical margins (*red arrow*). (C) Sagittal T2-weighted image shows hyperintense T2 signal filling the disk space (*red arrow*), as well as subjacent vertebral body bone marrow edema (*green arrow*). (D) Sagittal T1-weighted contrast-enhanced image shows peripheral enhancement of the disk (*green arrow*) and adjacent marrow, as well as the paraspinal tissues with epidural extension (*red arrow*).

Box 1
Causes of negative spine biopsy in the evaluation of postoperative spine infection

Concurrent antibiotic therapy

Insufficient specimen

Improper specimen handling and processing

Sampling of inappropriate or incorrect site

Lavage aspiration only

No vertebral endplate samples

should be carefully reviewed before the biopsy procedure to identify the most optimal sites for sampling, the correct spine level(s), and the optimal approach. These procedures can be performed with various forms of anesthesia. Postoperative spine patients are already uncomfortable from their previous surgery, and hence, due consideration ought to be given to using intravenous anesthesia or moderate sedation and analgesia. Spine biopsy can be performed with fluoroscopic or CT guidance. The procedure should be performed with strict aseptic technique to prevent contamination of the specimen or infection of a noninfected postoperative spine. Although the initial impulse of many operators is to just obtain fluid, usually by performing a lavage with a small-gauge spinal needle, the objective of the biopsy procedure should be to obtain tissue. This tissue consists of disk material, endplate samples, and inflamed paraspinal soft tissue. Therefore, the operator should have various biopsy needles available to perform the procedure. The tools should include not only small-gauge spinal needles but also soft tissue cutting or core needles, and bone biopsy needles. Many of the current biopsy systems can be deployed through coaxial techniques, which enhance the safety of these procedures and facilitate patient comfort. It is advisable to obtain as many specimens as possible, but no fewer than 3, for microbiological analysis. Disk material is difficult to aspirate with small-gauge needles. An automated percutaneous diskectomy device can be used to obtain adequate amounts of disk material.[25] Alternatively, a disk endplate biopsy can be performed to obtain several cores of bone from the vertebral body endplate. Specimens are submitted in sterile containers for microbiological analysis, including Gram stain, acid-fast stain, fungal smears, and culture. In addition, soft tissue and bone cores are submitted to surgical pathology for tissue analysis for the presence of inflammatory cells or granuloma formation.

Surgical intervention is generally indicated in patients with clinical and imaging evidence of progressive infection despite appropriate antibiotic therapy, deformity secondary to destruction of the vertebral bodies, or spinal cord impingement resulting in neurologic deficits caused by epidural abscess.[5] The most common cause of epidural abscess formation is direct extension from adjacent spondylodiskitis. The predominant pathogen associated with epidural abscess in nearly every collective study is *Staphylococcus aureus*, whereas coagulase-negative *Staphylococcus* is most commonly isolated among patients with spinal instrumentation.[26–29] Epidural abscess formation primarily develops in the thoracic and lumbar areas of the spinal cord, where the epidural space is comparatively larger and contains a higher volume of fat tissue.[26,27] A primary risk factor for infection is a history of diabetes mellitus.[27,30] In addition, patients with a compromised immune system, such as individuals positive for the human immunodeficiency virus, intravenous drug abusers, or those undergoing immunosuppressive therapy, are also at a significantly higher risk of postoperative spine infection.[30] Initially, epidural spread of infection may appear as nonspecific inflammatory soft tissue mass, or phlegmon showing hypointense signal on T1-weighted and hyperintense signal on T2-weighted imaging, with associated heterogeneous enhancement (**Fig. 3**). These findings may be difficult to distinguish from granulation tissue. As infected fluid accumulates within the epidural space, MR imaging shows isointense or hypointense signal relative to the spinal cord on T1-weighted images and high signal intensity with peripherally enhancing inflammatory tissue, compatible with epidural abscess formation.

The treatment of choice for postoperative spine epidural abscess focuses on removal of the infection through surgical decompression and drainage with systemic antibiotic therapy.[31] Conservative treatment has been implemented with some success in patients with small abscesses and is also used in patients who are not surgical candidates or those with advanced neurologic deficits that are deemed unlikely to improve with surgery.[31,32] Rarely, progression of an epidural abscess can cause compression and thrombophlebitis of the epidural veins, with the possibility of spinal cord infarct. Thus, delays in diagnosis and surgical intervention can result in irreversible neurologic spinal cord injury.[27,28,33,34] If MR imaging is contraindicated, CT myelography shows blockage of normal flowing contrast at the level of extradural compression, from either an epidural inflammatory process or abscess.

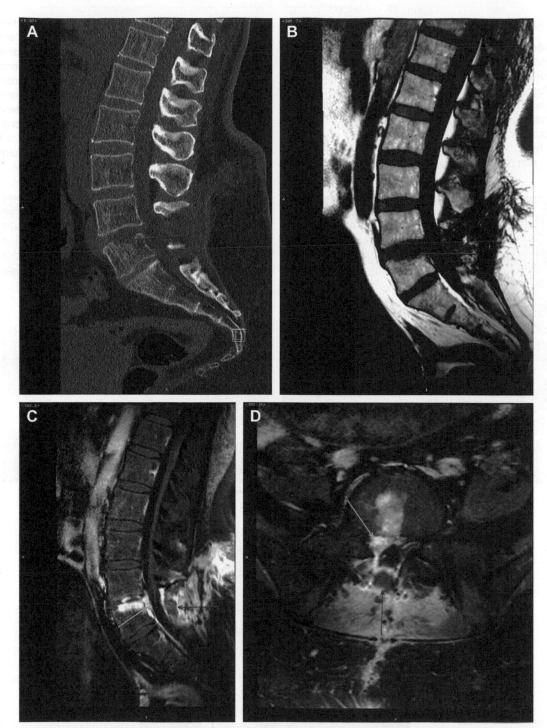

Fig. 3. Septic spondylodiskitis with epidural abscess. Patient is 1 month status after L4-L5 laminectomy and partial diskectomy. (*A*) Reformatted sagittal CT image shows irregularity and erosion of the cortical bone along the superior endplate of L5 (*red arrow*). (*B*) Sagittal T1-weighted MR image shows loss of the normal hypointense band of cortical bone (*red arrow*). (*C*) Sagittal and (*D*) axial contrast-enhanced MR images demonstrate epidural soft tissue lesions and enhancement, as well as rimlike enhancement of a paraspinal abscess (*red arrow*) and phlegmonous epidural (*green arrow*) and paravertebral enhancement.

PARAVERTEBRAL ABSCESS

After spine surgery, infiltrative edema and enhancement are commonly identified in the paravertebral soft tissues and epidural space. Postoperative fluid collections are commonly identified, such as seroma, hematoma, or pseudomeningocele, and must be differentiated from infected collections (**Fig. 4**).[2] Contiguous spread of infection from the spine to adjacent soft tissues, or hematogenous spread via paravertebral veins, can result in paravertebral or psoas abscess formation. The lower thoracic or lumbar regions are more often affected. The cause in postoperative spine patients is often bacterial. If the vertebral infection spreads to adjacent vascular structures, it can rarely lead to the development of mycotic aneurysms, which has high mortality.[35–39] Similar to epidural or intervertebral disk space collections, paravertebral abscesses show hypointense T1 and hyperintense T2 signal with irregular

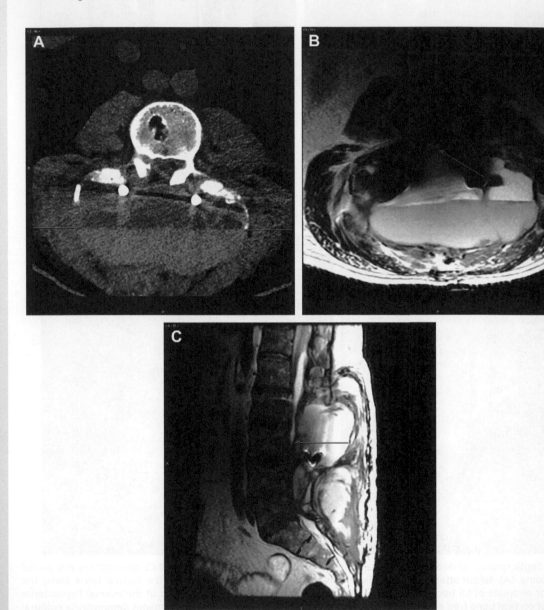

Fig. 4. Infected postoperative hematoma. Patient 1 month status after multilevel laminectomy and fusion. (*A*) Axial CT image shows a large posterior fluid collection with a hematocrit level, the denser independent portion representing blood clot (*red arrows*). (*B*) Axial and (*C*) sagittal T2-weighted images show the fluid-fluid level in the collection, which surrounds the posterior spinal fusion hardware and extends into the epidural space compressing the thecal sac (*red arrow*).

enhancing thick walls. Small paravertebral or psoas abscesses may respond to medical management; however, larger collections usually require CT-guided aspiration and drainage.[40]

SUMMARY

Imaging evaluation of postoperative spinal infection is challenging. A systematic approach and keen understanding of multimodality imaging techniques, as well as the knowledge of the patient's surgical procedure and clinical presentation, are critical for the radiologist to render an accurate diagnosis. Because of the overlap between diagnostic imaging findings in the postoperative spine and the infected spine, in those situations in which the index of clinical suspicion for spine infection is high, then immediate consideration ought to be given to performing a spine biopsy.

REFERENCES

1. Vertinsky A, Krasnokutsky M, Augustin M, et al. Cutting-edge imaging of the spine. Spinal imaging: overview and update. Neuroimaging Clin N Am 2007;17(1):117–36.
2. Hankcock C, Quencer R, Falcone S. Challenges and pitfalls in postoperative spine imaging. Applied Radiology 2008;37(2):23–34.
3. Weinstein MA, McCabe JP, Cammisa FP. Postoperative spinal wound infection: a review of 2391 consecutive index procedures. J Spinal Disord 2000;13:422–6.
4. Chaudhary SB, Vivies MJ, Basra SK, et al. Postoperative spinal wound infections and postprocedural diskitis. J Spinal Cord Med 2007;30(5):441–51.
5. Hegde V, Meredith DS, Kepler CK, et al. Management of postoperative spinal infections. World J Orthop 2012;3(11):182–9.
6. Berquist T. Imaging of the postoperative spine. Radiol Clin North Am 2006;44(3):407–18.
7. Douglas-Akinwande AC, Buckwalter KA, Rydberg J, et al. Multichannel CT: evaluating the spine in postoperative patients with orthopedic hardware. Radiographics 2006;26(Suppl 1):S97–110.
8. Hayashi D, Roemer FW, Mian A, et al. Imaging features of postoperative complications after spinal surgery and instrumentation. AJR Am J Roentgenol 2012;199(1):W123–9.
9. Thakkar RS, Malloy JP, Thakkar SC, et al. Imaging the postoperative spine. Radiol Clin North Am 2012;50(4):731–47.
10. Rutherford EE, Tarplett LJ, Davies EM, et al. Lumbar spine fusion and stabilization: hardware, techniques, and imaging appearances. Radiographics 2007;27(6):1737–49.
11. Stradiotti P, Curti A, Castellazzi G, et al. Metal-related artifacts in instrumented spine. Techniques for reducing artifacts in CT and MRI: state of the art. Eur Spine J 2009;18(Suppl 1):102–8.
12. Palestro CJ, Torres MA. Radionuclide imaging in orthopedic infections. Semin Nucl Med 1997;27:334–45.
13. Love C, Patel M, Lonner BS, et al. Diagnosing spinal osteomyelitis: a comparison of bone and Ga-67 scintigraphy and magnetic resonance imaging. Clin Nucl Med 2000;25:963–77.
14. Gratz S, Dörner J, Fischer U, et al. 18F-FDG hybrid PET in patients with suspected spondylitis. Eur J Nucl Med Mol Imaging 2002;29:516–24.
15. Gouliouris T, Aliyu SH, Brown NM. Spondylodiscitis: update on diagnosis and management. J Antimicrob Chemother 2010;65(Suppl 3):iii11–24.
16. Silber JS, Anderson DG, Vaccaro AR, et al. NASS management of postprocedural discitis. Spine J 2002;2(4):279–87.
17. Lazennec JY, Fourniols E, Lenoir T, et al. Infections in the operated spine: update on risk management and therapeutic strategies. Orthop Traumatol Surg Res 2011;97(Suppl 6):S107–16.
18. Go JL, Rothman S, Prosper A, et al. Spine infections. Neuroimaging Clin N Am 2012;22(4):755–72.
19. Van Goethem JW, Parizel PM, Jinkins JR. Review article: MRI of the postoperative lumbar spine. Neuroradiology 2002;44:723–39.
20. Bommireddy R, Kamat A, Smith ET, et al. Magnetic resonance image findings in the early postoperative period after anterior cervical discectomy. Eur Spine J 2007;16(1):27–31.
21. Tali ET. Spinal infections. Eur J Radiol 2004;50:120–33.
22. Ledermann HP, Schweitzer ME, Morrison WB, et al. MR imaging findings in spinal infections: rules or myths? Radiology 2003;228(2):506–14.
23. Eguchi Y, Ohtori S, Yamashita M, et al. Diffusion magnetic resonance imaging to differentiate degenerative from infectious endplate abnormalities in the lumbar spine. Spine 2011;36(3):E198–202.
24. Michel SC, Pfirrmann CW, Boos N, et al. CT-guided core biopsy of subchondral bone and intervertebral space in suspected spondylodiskitis. AJR Am J Roentgenol 2006;186(4):977–80.
25. Wattamwar A, Ortiz OA. Use of a percutaneous diskectomy device to facilitate the diagnosis of infectious spondylitis. AJNR Am J Neuroradiol 2010;31:1157–8.
26. Danner RL, Hartman BJ. Update on spinal epidural abscess: 35 cases and review of the literature. Rev Infect Dis 1987;9(2):265–74.
27. Hlavin ML, Kaminski HJ, Ross JS, et al. Spinal epidural abscess: a ten-year perspective. Neurosurgery 1990;27(2):177–84.

28. Nussbaum ES, Rigamonti D, Standiford H, et al. Spinal epidural abscess: a report of 40 cases and review. Surg Neurol 1992;38(3):225–31.

29. Rigamonti D, Liem L, Wolf AL, et al. Epidural abscess in the cervical spine. Mt Sinai J Med 1994; 61(4):357–62.

30. Reihsaus EH, Waldbaur W. Spinal epidural abscess: a meta-analysis of 915 patients. Neurosurg Rev 2000;23(4):175–204 [discussion: 205].

31. Rigamonti D, Liem L, Sampath P, et al. Spinal epidural abscess: contemporary trends in etiology, evaluation, and management. Surg Neurol 1999; 52(2):189–96 [discussion: 197].

32. Khanna RK, Malik GM, Rock JP, et al. Spinal epidural abscess: evaluation of factors influencing outcome. Neurosurgery 1996;39(5):958–64.

33. Grewal S, Hocking G, Wildsmith JA. Epidural abscesses. Br J Anaesth 2006;96(3):292–302.

34. Darouiche RO. Spinal epidural abscess. N Engl J Med 2006;355(19):2012–20.

35. Chen SH, Lin WC, Lee CH, et al. Spontaneous infective spondylitis and mycotic aneurysm: incidence, risk factors, outcome and management experience. Eur Spine J 2008;17(3):439–44.

36. Dahl T, Lange C, Ødegård A, et al. Ruptured abdominal aortic aneurysm secondary to tuberculous spondylitis. Int Angiol 2005;24(1):98–101.

37. Lifeso RM, Weaver P, Harder EH. Tuberculous spondylitis in adults. J Bone Joint Surg Am 1985;67(9): 1405–13.

38. Winkler S, Wiesinger E, Graninger W. Extrapulmonary tuberculosis with paravertebral abscess formation and thyroid involvement. Infection 1994;22(6):420–2.

39. Gonda RL, Gutierrez OH, Azodo MV. Mycotic aneurysms of the aorta: radiologic features. Radiology 1988;168(2):343–6.

40. Pull ter Gunne AF, Mohamed AS, Skolasky RL, et al. The presentation, incidence, etiology, and treatment of surgical site infections after spinal surgery. Spine (Phila Pa 1976) 2010;35(13):1323–8.

Radiologic Evaluation and Management of Postoperative Spine Paraspinal Fluid Collections

Nikhil K. Jain, MD, MBA[a], Kimberly Dao, MD[b],
A. Orlando Ortiz, MD, MBA[a,*]

KEYWORDS

- Postoperative spine • Seroma • Hematoma • Pseudomeningocele • Abscess

KEY POINTS

- Paraspinal fluid collections are often seen after spine surgery. This increased frequency is likely due to surgical manipulation, but may also reflect other factors such as the extent of the spine surgery, patient comorbidities, and patient coagulation status.
- Postoperative imaging modalities include myelography, ultrasound, radionuclide scanning, computed tomographic scan, and magnetic resonance imaging. Magnetic resonance imaging remains the best study to visualize and define the spectrum of paraspinal fluid collections.
- Management of paraspinal fluid collections is challenging. Communication between the radiologist and surgeon is extremely helpful in managing these complex situations.

INTRODUCTION

The high prevalence of back and/or neck pain in the United States population is estimated at 20%.[1] A large number of these patients initially or eventually undergo spinal surgery. Approximately 1.2 million spine surgeries, including 300,000 spinal fusion surgeries, are performed each year in the United States.[2] It is always important to try to understand why an operative intervention was performed. The indications for spine surgery include deformity correction for congenital scoliosis, relief of neural compression from space-occupying lesions such as disc herniation, osteophyte formation, epidural mass or hematoma, relief of spinal canal stenosis due to degenerative or infectious spine disease, or correction of spinal instability.[3] This information may be helpful in understanding why a potential complication occurs.

For example, an analysis of non-neurologic complications following spinal surgery for adolescent idiopathic scoliosis in 702 patients showed that hematoma, seroma, and dehiscence occurred in 0.71% of the surgeries. These latter complications were associated with increased blood loss and prolonged operative and anesthesia times.[4] In addition, knowledge of the specific type of spinal surgery, whether it is deconstructive such as a laminectomy for spinal stenosis or reconstructive such as a fusion for instability, can be helpful in the search for abnormal paraspinal fluid collections. The radiologist should be familiar with the types of surgical approaches, tools, implants, and techniques associated with spine surgeries as this will assist in identifying focal abnormalities. Approaches may consist of anterior, posterior, or combined anterior-posterior and may use

Disclosures: None.
[a] Department of Radiology, Winthrop-University Hospital, 259 First Street, Mineola, NY 11501, USA; [b] Division of Internal Medicine, University of Pittsburgh Medical Center, Montefiore Hospital, 3 West 933, 200 Lothrop Street, Pittsburgh, PA 15213, USA
* Corresponding author.
E-mail address: oortiz@winthrop.org

instrumentation such as screws, spinal wires, artificial ligaments, vertebral cages, artificial discs, and osteoinductive agents.[5] Different spine fusion techniques are associated with different complications and complication rates.[6]

Although most spine surgeries are successful, complications may be observed. Postoperative spine paraspinal fluid collections are not uncommon. They may or may not be symptomatic, but their presence, either as an incidental finding or as a possible etiologic agent in the postoperative patient's clinical presentation, requires careful evaluation and management. Given their frequent occurrence, they have received limited attention in the medical literature, yet often pose a diagnostic dilemma for both surgeon and radiologist alike. The purpose of this article is to describe the various types of paraspinal postoperative fluid collections with respect to their imaging findings,

to characterize them, and to suggest possible management strategies.

Different types of fluid collections may be encountered within or about the spinal axis following spine surgery. Fortunately, the overwhelming majority of these collections are self-limited and resolve with conservative management. There are those paraspinal fluid collections, however, that are found on postoperative spine imaging evaluation in symptomatic patients that may require further diagnostic evaluation, such as percutaneous aspiration, or additional surgical intervention such as open decompression and/or medical management with prolonged antibiotic therapy (Fig. 1). The fluid collections may be classified by location, intra-spinal or within the epidural compartment, or paraspinal, that is anterior, dorsal, or lateral to the spinal axis. These collections may also be classified by type and

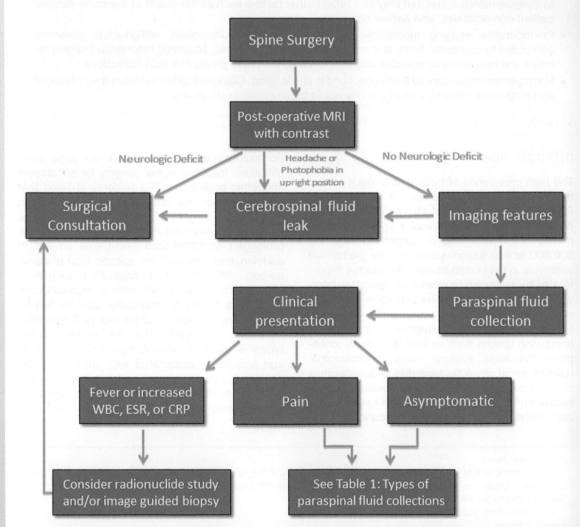

Fig. 1. Diagnostic algorithm for management of postoperative spine paraspinal fluid collections. CRP, C-reactive protein; ESR, erythrocyte sedimentation rate; WBC, white blood cell count.

Table 1
Types of paraspinal fluid collections and their locations

Hematoma	Intraspinal, paraspinal
Seroma	Paraspinal
Pseudomeningocoele	Paraspinal
Abscess	Intraspinal, paraspinal

include hematoma, seroma, pseudomeningocele, and abscess (**Table 1**). It is very important for the radiologist to be aware of when the surgical procedure was performed, not only to better understand the imaging manifestations of the collection, but also to determine whether prior preoperative and postoperative imaging examinations are available for comparison. Hematomas may be seen acutely after spine surgery; abscesses may be seen subacutely, and seromas and pseudomeningoceles may be seen as subacute or chronic processes.[3]

HEMATOMA

A hematoma is an extravascular collection of blood of variable size and extent that can, postsurgically, occur within or outside of the spinal canal. These focal hemorrhages may result from surgical manipulation and damage to blood vessels in the operative field. They are uncommon and occur in less than 1% of spine surgery patients, in 5.4% of patients undergoing posterior lumbar fusion, and in 5.6% of anterior cervical discectomy and fusion cases.[6–8] Patients with coagulation deficits, either intrinsic or related to anticoagulation medication, or with multilevel spine surgery, may also be at increased risk for developing postsurgical

hematomas.[2,8] Hematomas occur acutely and, depending on the size, location, and extent of the hemorrhage, can present in the acute or early subacute postsurgical period. The clinical presentation may occur within hours to days after spine surgery.[7,9] Patients may present with increasing, severe sharp pain with or without a radiating component.[9] Patients may also present with focal neurologic deficits especially when the hematoma is located in the epidural space.[2] It is therefore essential to perform an imaging study urgently in a postoperative spine patient with this type of clinical presentation (**Table 2**). Anterior paraspinal hematomas may compress the upper aerodigestive tract, resulting in dysphagia and/or respiratory distress.[3]

The imaging study of choice to evaluate a patient with a suspected hematoma in the epidural space is magnetic resonance (MR) imaging. The MR imaging appearance of an acute epidural hematoma is that of a somewhat heterogeneous hypointense to isointense fluid collection on T1-weighted sequences and a heterogeneous hypointense to hyperintense fluid collection on T2-weighted sequences. Gradient echo sequences may show foci of hypointensity. Delayed hematomas may show increased signal intensity on both T1-weighted and T2-weighted images.[9] If present within the epidural space, the collection may extend for several vertebral body segments and may be associated with spinal cord impingement and spinal cord edema (**Fig. 2**). Hematomas that are located outside of the spinal canal, within or adjacent to the paraspinal muscles, may show signal changes on T1-weighted and T2-weighted sequences that parallel the evolution of blood breakdown products.[10] Indeed, over time, a hematocrit level may be seen, such that with more chronic hematomas, it may be impossible to

Table 2
Postoperative spine hematoma

Definition	A contained intraspinal and/or paraspinal hemorrhagic collection that can be found anywhere along the course of the operative tract
Imaging findings	Acute: hyperdense to isodense on CT; hypointense to isointense on T1 and heterogeneously hypointense to hyperintense on T2 MR imaging; mild peripheral enhancement on MR imaging Subacute: hypodense on CT; increased signal intensity on T1 and T2; mild peripheral enhancement; hematocrit level may be present on either study Chronic: hypodense on CT; fluid signal on T1 and T2 MR imaging with residual foci of low high signal on T1 and low signal on T2
Management	Asymptomatic patient: observation and imaging surveillance Symptomatic patient: Epidural hematoma: surgical consultation for probable evacuation Paraspinal: image-guided percutaneous or surgical drainage

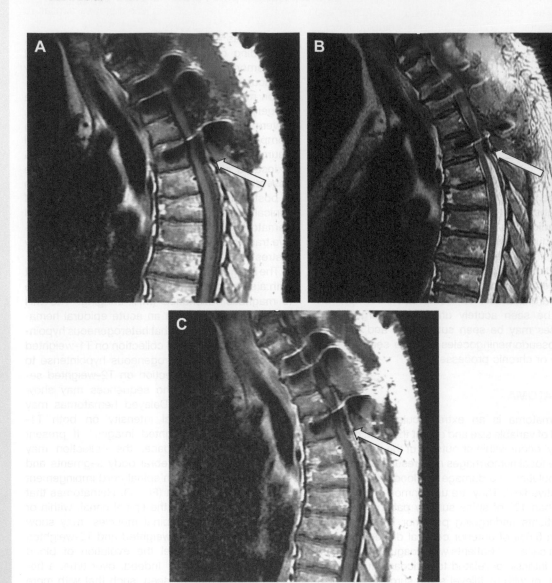

Fig. 2. Severe back pain status post recent thoracic posterior instrumentation. Sagittal T1-weighted (*A*), T2-weighted (*B*), and contrast-enhanced T1-weighted (*C*) MR images demonstrate a dorsal epidural fluid collection in the upper thoracic spine with effacement of the dorsal subarachnoid space and encroachment on the spinal cord. The collection (*arrow*) is predominantly hypointense on T1-weighted (*A*) and T2-weighted (*B*) images with enhancement of the adjacent dura (*C*) and is consistent with an acute epidural hematoma. (*Courtesy of* Dr Jeffrey Ross, MD, Barrow Neurological Institute, Phoenix, AZ.)

distinguish them from seromas (**Fig. 3**). Thin peripheral contrast enhancement may be observed. On computed tomographic scan (CT), hematomas, depending on their age and location, will manifest as increased, intermediate, or low attenuation. They can be difficult to detect in the acute phase, as the attenuation may be comparable with that of other adjacent soft tissue structures.

Epidural hematomas often require immediate surgical consideration for evacuation. A large epidural hematoma in a symptomatic patient will likely require surgical decompression with laminectomy and removal of the hematoma. Smaller and more chronic-appearing epidural or paraspinal hematomas are often managed conservatively and may require imaging surveillance to assess for any interval change in size and appearance.[11] In asymptomatic patients with chronic-appearing small (less than one vertebral segment) hematomas or seromas that are gradually involuting, it may be prudent to avoid percutaneous aspiration as this procedure may predispose to superinfection of a sterile collection. Percutaneous aspiration of paraspinal hematomas may be

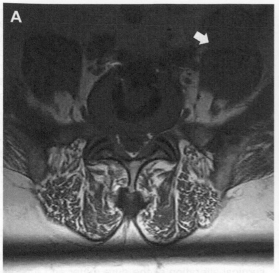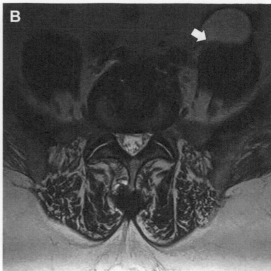

Fig. 3. A 60-year-old man with prior anterior lumbar interbody fusion and low back pain. Axial T1-weighted (*A*) and T2-weighted (*B*) MR images demonstrate a well-defined fluid collection along the anterior aspect of left psoas muscle with T1- and T2-hypointense signal and a fluid–fluid level (*arrow*) compatible with subacute/resolving hematoma.

considered in patients in whom symptoms may be referable to the collection or in whom the collection is already suspected to be infected. In this situation, the procedure should be performed with strict aseptic technique with subsequent careful monitoring and follow-up of the patient. Hematomas in the subdural space following spine surgery are rare and more often associated with procedures such as lumbar puncture or spinal anesthesia.[2]

SEROMA

A seroma is a fluid collection that contains lymphatic fluid and may or may not be surrounded by a fibrous capsule. The presence of a seroma reflects disruption of local lymphatic vessels.[12] Given the close proximity of lymphatics to arterial, capillary, and venous structures, it is not uncommon to have some disruption of these structures during surgery and to have a relatively lesser amount of hemorrhage accumulate within the seroma as well. This accumulation of hemorrhage may result in a hematocrit level within the seroma and may account for the overlap in the literature with respect to classification; seromas and hematomas are often considered similar entities. Seromas can be located anywhere along the path of surgical intervention and may be seen subcutaneously or adjacent to the spinal canal or paraspinal soft tissue structures. Postoperative spine seromas are to be distinguished from Morel-Lavallee seromas; the latter are seen after blunt closed soft tissue trauma or after abdominal reconstructive or plastic surgery.[12] The Morel-Lavallee seromas are located subcutaneously and often respond to treatment with compression bandages (**Table 3**).

Table 3 Postoperative spine seroma	
Definition	A fluid collection that contains lymphatic fluid and may or may not be surrounded by a fibrous capsule
Imaging findings	CT: hypodense paraspinal fluid collection; MR imaging: fluid signal on T1-, T2-, and diffusion-weighted images. Mild peripheral enhancement on MR imaging. A small amount of debris or hemorrhage may layer dependently within the collection
Management	Small seromas tend to be asymptomatic and can be observed Larger seromas can be associated with symptoms Treatment options: compression bandages, image-guided percutaneous or surgical drainage, especially when possibility of infection is clinically suspected

The true incidence of seromas is unknown, but the incidence among posterior fusion surgeries is up to 5.4% when grouped with hematomas.[6] Experiences with osteoinductive agents like recombinant human bone mineral protein (rhBMP-2) have shown an increased incidence of painful seromas,[13] which suggests that an inflammatory response may play a role in seroma formation.[14,15] Bone mineral proteins are associated with inflammatory reactions in other structures, such as joints and blood vessels. In a study of 234 patients who underwent anterior cervical fusion with and without rhBMP-2, 27.5% of the group that received rhBMP-2 experienced significant swelling versus 3.6% of the group that did not receive the agent.[16] Another study in which rhBMP-2 was used in posterolateral fusion of 140 patients showed a 4.6% incidence of edema with seroma formation.[13] In a large series involving the use of bone mineral protein in posterior spinal fusion, a 2.8% rate of seroma formation associated with nerve root compression was observed.[17] On the other hand, seromas have been observed in the absence of bone mineral protein use. The type of surgical procedure may predispose a patient to seroma formation as there is an increased association between posterior lumbar fusion (posterolateral, posterior lumber interbody, transforaminal) for spondylolisthesis and subsequent seroma formation.[6]

The imaging findings in patients with seromas are dependent on the size, location, and age of the fluid collection. Plain radiography, rarely, may demonstrate a focal soft tissue density. An ultrasound examination may reveal either an anechoic or a hypoechoic paraspinal fluid collection; the presence of increased echogenicity suggests the presence of a hemorrhagic component. On unenhanced CT examinations, seromas present as hypodense focal paraspinal fluid collections that are located in close proximity to the site of surgical intervention. A small hematocrit level may be present. MR imaging shows low T1 and increased T2 signal intensity within a focal fluid collection (**Fig. 4**). A small hematocrit level may also be observed on MR imaging; the signal characteristics of the dependent aspect of the collection will depend on the age of the seroma. The margin of the seroma may show uniform wall enhancement following the administration of an intravenous gadolinium contrast agent.[12] The presence of a capsule may have implications for subsequent management: encapsulated and symptomatic seromas may require surgical excision, whereas unencapsulated seromas can be treated with compression bandages or percutaneous drainage.[12] Percutaneous aspiration of a seroma may be indicated in situations whereby a symptomatic postoperative spine patient presents with a paraspinal fluid collection that may represent a seroma, abscess, cystic portion of a previously resected cystic mass, or an acquired meningocele (**Fig. 5**). Percutaneous image-guided techniques may also be used to drain the seroma or to place a drainage catheter, such as a hemovac drain, into a large collection.[13] In patients in whom the use of a bone mineral protein is anticipated, Shahlaie and Kim[15] advocate the use of fibrin glue to surround the rhBMP-2 or to consider the use of perioperative steroids.

PSEUDOMENINGOCELE

A postoperative pseudomeningocele is a collection of cerebrospinal fluid that, as a result of surgical alteration of the dura mater and the surrounding osseous structures or laminae, extends from the spinal canal into the adjacent paraspinal soft tissues.[10] These postoperative pseudomeningoceles are to be distinguished from post-traumatic pseudomeningoceles of the exiting spinal nerve roots, based upon location and etiology. The margins of the postsurgical pseudomeningocele are comprised of reactive fibrous tissue and not the meninges.[10] This contrasts with true meningoceles, which are dural-lined cerebrospinal fluid containing fluid collections that extend through an osseous defect in the craniospinal axis and present as congenital lesions or in association with connective tissue disorders, such as neurofibromatosis type 1, homocystinuria, Marfan or Ehlers-Danlos syndromes. Pseudomeningoceles are not uncommon and have a reported incidence of 0.068% to 2%.[18] These collections are seen in up to 2% of patients undergoing lumbar laminectomy.[2] The true incidence of postoperative pseudomeningoceles is not known as these collections are often asymptomatic.[18] Pseudomeningoceles develop after surgical laceration of the dura mater and other meningeal layers during surgery or following incomplete closure of the meninges in the case of intradural surgery.[10] The incidence of incidental durotomy occurs in 1% to 15.9% of spine surgeries, with the greatest incidence seen in patients undergoing revision spine surgery.[8] Most durotomies are recognized and repaired at the time of the surgical procedure. In those that go unrecognized, however, due to resulting meningeal defect, cerebrospinal fluid leaks into the adjacent paraspinal soft tissue space and is associated with a fibrous soft tissue reaction that gradually confines the cerebrospinal fluid. These fluid collections can range in size from 1 to 10 cm.[2] Pseudomeningoceles are most often

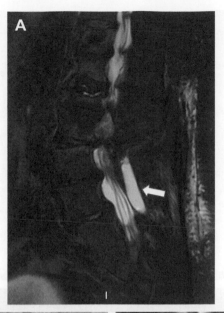

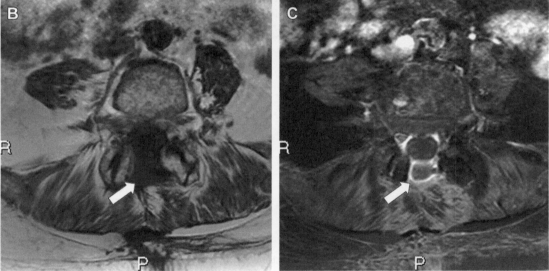

Fig. 4. An 85-year-old woman status post L3-5 laminectomy for spinal canal decompression 1 year before this study, with low back pain due to an L1 vertebral compression fracture. Fat-suppressed sagittal T2-weighted MR image (A) shows a 4.8-cm fluid collection at the L3-5 laminectomy site compatible with postoperative seroma. Note prior T11 vertebral augmentation and acute L2 superior endplate fracture with a cleft. T1-weighted axial (B) and fat-suppressed T1-weighted axial contrast-enhanced (C) images show a 1.3 × 1.1-cm fluid collection with enhancing margins at the laminectomy site (arrow).

found at the level of the lumbar spine, adjacent to a laminectomy site and dorsal to the thecal sac. Their preponderance in the lumbar spine may reflect a combination of several factors, including the increased frequency of lumbar spine surgeries as well as the possibility of greater hydrostatic pressure in the lumbar spinal canal as compared to other levels of the spinal axis.[18,19] Indeed, pseudomeningoceles are seen in patients who have

undergone prior lumbar laminectomy for either lumbar stenosis or lumbar disc surgery, including discectomy and resection of herniated disc fragments.[2,10]

The majority of pseudomeningoceles are asymptomatic.[18] These collections, however, can be associated with axial low back pain, radicular pain, or headache, including postural headache. Pseudomeningoceles may compress adjacent

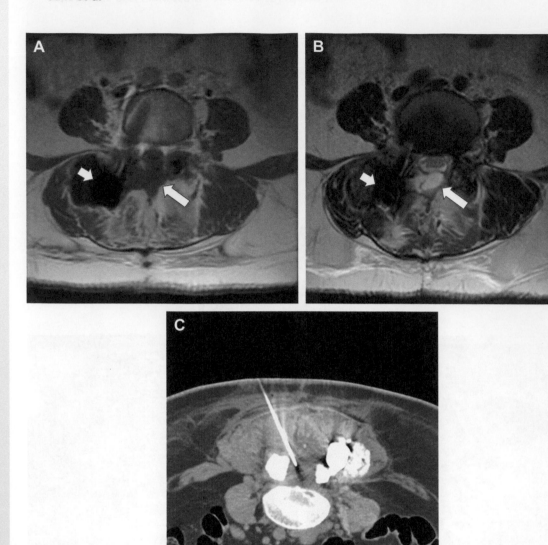

Fig. 5. A 48-year-old woman status post L4-5 laminectomy with transpedicular fixation. T1- (*A*) and T2- (*B*) weighted axial MR images show a fluid collection in the laminectomy bed compatible with seroma mildly compressing the thecal sac (*long arrow*). Note the right-sided transpedicular screw (*short arrow*). Axial CT image (*C*) of the lumbar spine with the patient in the prone position shows needle placement into the seroma for aspiration; the fluid analysis was unremarkable.

nerve roots or may be associated with periradicular fibrosis and adhesions.[2] Large pseudomeningoceles may extend to the skin surface where they present as fluctuant subcutaneous masses (**Figs. 6** and **7**). The proximity to a postsurgical wound may predispose these latter types of collections to superinfection with the subsequent development of meningitis and/or abscess formation. The pseudomeningocele may also form a cutaneous fistula resulting in a cerebrospinal fluid leak (**Fig. 8**).

On imaging, pseudomeningoceles present as irregular, lobulated, or oblong fluid collections that are located adjacent to a laminectomy site. The fluid collection demonstrates the imaging characteristics of cerebrospinal fluid on all imaging modalities including ultrasound, CT, and MR imaging. The collection is located adjacent to the thecal sac and laminectomy defects and/or surgical hardware are often present. It is important to visualize the full extent of the collection on the imaging study. If there has been prior spine

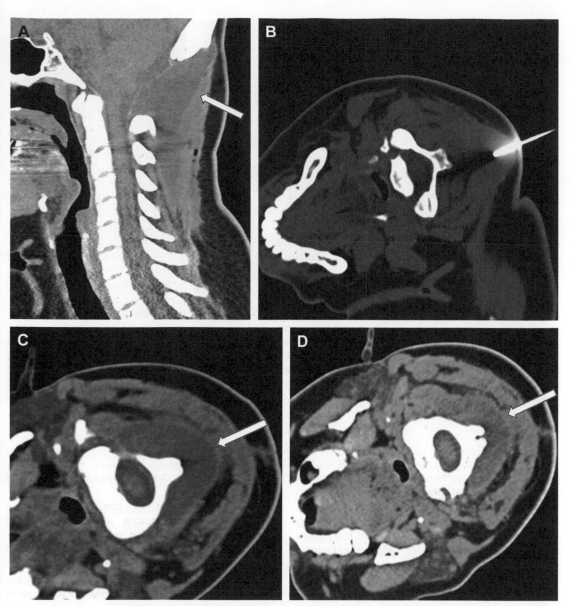

Fig. 6. A 46-year-old woman status post surgical decompression with suboccipital craniectomy for Chiari I malformation and cervical syringohydromyelia. Sagittal 2-dimensional CT reformation of the cervical spine (*A*) shows a large posterior cervical space midline fluid collection at the level of the posterior craniocervical junction with deep and superficial components compatible with pseudomeningocele (*arrow*). Axial cervical spine CT image (*B*) with patient in the decubitus position shows a spinal needle placed into the fluid collection. Axial cervical spine CT image shows the fluid collection preaspiration (*C*) and partial resolution of the fluid collection after aspiration of 25 mL of clear slightly straw-colored fluid (*D*) (*arrow*). The remainder of the collection resorbed after application of a compression bandage with no subsequent reaccumulation of fluid.

instrumentation, then the relationship of the collection to the spinal hardware should be fully characterized; this may be difficult, however, due to the imaging artifacts associated with spine hardware on both CT and MR imaging. The dorsal extent of the collection should also be defined relative to the skin surface and to the site of surgery. On CT, the collection is hypodense, often isodense to cerebrospinal fluid. In specific instances, especially when the patient cannot undergo an MR imaging examination or where there is a suspicion of cerebrospinal fluid leak, a spinal

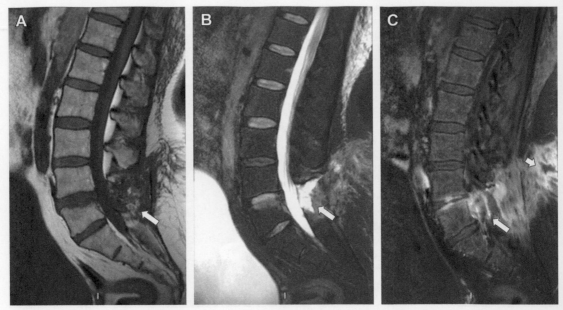

Fig. 7. A 50-year-old woman status post L4-5 and L5-S1 laminectomy for spinal canal decompression and L4-5 discectomy and pseudomeningocele formation. T1-weighted (*A*) and T2-weighted (*B*) sagittal MR images show a 2.0 × 2.6-cm fluid collection in the laminectomy bed at L4-5 with mild mass effect on the posterior aspect of the thecal sac (*arrow*). Fat-suppressed contrast-enhanced T1-weighted sagittal MR image (*C*) shows enhancement of the fluid collection with enhancement extending into L4-5 disc level (*long arrow*). The deep fluid collection is continuous with an enhancing fluid collection in the superficial subcutaneous tissues (*small arrow*).

puncture may be performed with the subsequent placement of an ntrathecal contrast agent and the performance of immediate and, possibly delayed, post-myelogram CT images. Depending on the size and extent of the dural tear, there may be either immediate or delayed leakage of contrast into the paraspinal collection. Pseudomeningoceles demonstrate cerebrospinal fluid signal intensity on T1-, T2-, and diffusion-weighted sequences; fluid-fluid levels, however, may also be seen due to the presence of post-surgical debris or blood products.[20] The presence of residual postsurgical hemorrhage may confound the MR imaging presentation.[21] The T2-weighted sequence, in sagittal and axial planes, may help to visualize the pseudomeningocele and its communications.[2] On MR imaging, pseudomeningoceles may show mild enhancement along their margins and near the laminectomy site following intravenous contrast administration. Increased or more prominent contrast enhancement should raise the possibility of infection. In patients with active cerebrospinal fluid leaks, the presence of prominent dural enhancement may be suggestive of cerebrospinal fluid hypotension. The precise location

of the dural tear may not always be identified with imaging.[20]

The management of pseudomeningoceles depends on many factors, especially size and symptomatic presentation. In general, small asymptomatic pseudomeningoceles are observed and not treated. These small pseudomeningoceles gradually resolve over time.[18,22] Regardless of size, pseudomeningoceles that present shortly after surgery with a cerebrospinal fluid fistula may benefit from the placement of either a blood patch or a spine drain.[2,18] Pseudomeningoceles that are associated with symptoms weeks to months after the initial spine surgical procedure may require direct surgical repair of the dural defect. In these latter patients, subarachnoid drain placement aids in the formation of seal at the leakage site and increases healing by cerebrospinal fluid diversion.[18] Large pseudomeningoceles may also require primary closure with patch techniques using autologous tissue, dural allografts, or fibrin glue along the suture line. In those cases where dural adhesions are present, release of the entrapped neural element (nerve root or spinal cord) can be performed (**Table 4**).[18]

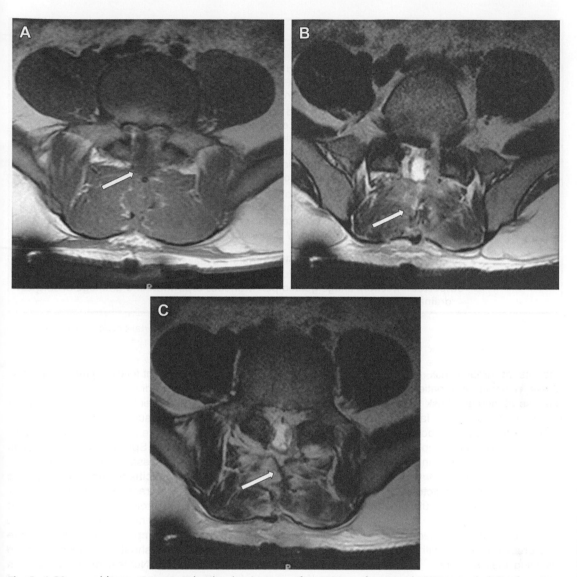

Fig. 8. A 30-year-old man status post lumbar laminectomy for excision of a ventral L5-S1 extruded disc fragment with a cerebrospinal fluid leak. Axial T1- (*A*) and T2- (*B* and *C*) weighted MR images show a focal midline surgical defect that extends from the laminectomy site to skin surface (*arrow*).

ABSCESS

An abscess is a focal circumscribed infected fluid collection. Infection is an uncommon and undesirable complication of spine surgery. The overall incidence of postoperative spine infection ranges from 0.2% to 20%; the lower rate of spine infection is seen in patients who receive intravenous antibiotic prophylaxis within an hour of surgery.[2] The most common pathogen that is seen identified as the source of infection is *Staphylococcus aureus*. *Staphylococcus epidermidis* and *Propionibacterium acnes* are common pathogens

associated with implant infections.[23] Multiple factors may predispose the postoperative spine patient to infection. First, contamination of the operative site may occur before, during, or just after the surgical procedure. Presurgical infection may be seen with pre-existing occult infections that subsequently spread to the surgical site. Surgical dissection results in the creation of potential avascularized dead spaces in the operative bed, which may serve as sites for potential microbial growth. Specific host factors include patient age and comorbidities, with elderly and debilitated

Table 4
Postoperative spine pseudomeningocele

Definition	A collection of cerebrospinal fluid that, as a result of surgical alteration of the dura mater and the surrounding osseous structures or laminae, extends from the spinal canal into the adjacent paraspinal soft tissues
Imaging findings	Predominantly cerebrospinal fluid attenuation on CT and signal intensity on MR imaging sequences; variable size and shape of collection that is contiguous with postsurgical site. Small fluid-fluid levels due to postsurgical hemorrhage into collection. Mild peripheral contrast enhancement on MR imaging; more intense enhancement should raise suspicion for possible infection. Dural enhancement may be seen in patients with cerebrospinal fluid hypotension
Management	Small, asymptomatic collections: observation Symptomatic collections (headache or pain), regardless of size, may require epidural blood patch or drainage catheter placement or surgical repair of the durotomy. More superficial collections may respond to drainage and/or application of pressure dressings Symptomatic collections with cerebrospinal fluid leak may require a spine drain and/or exploration and repair of the durotomy Suspected infection: image-guided percutaneous aspiration and drainage or surgical drainage with antibiotic therapy

patients at greater risk for infection. Morbidly obese patients and patients with incontinence are also at increased risk for postoperative spine infection. Intraoperative factors that may predispose a patient toward a postoperative spine infection include prolonged operation time, increased procedural blood loss, and increased number of operative levels. For example, the published rate of infection after discectomy is 0.6% to 3.7% compared with 3.7% to 20% after posterior instrumented fusion.[24]

Patients with postoperative spine infections may present clinically within 1 week to 4 months following their surgery.[7,24] Patients may present with increasing pain, low-grade fever, and/or with drainage from the surgical site. As these patients are often on analgesics, the temperature elevation may not be as apparent. Laboratory parameters that may be elevated include the white blood cell count, the erythrocyte sedimentation rate, and the C-reactive protein. Patients with suspected infection often undergo at least 2 imaging studies. In patients with an abscess, cross-sectional imaging with CT or MR imaging often shows an ill-defined fluid collection (**Fig. 9**). The collection is hypodense to isodense on CT. It is isointense to hypointense on T1-weighted images and hyperintense on T2-weighted images. The collection may demonstrate increased signal intensity on diffusion-weighted images with corresponding decreased signal intensity on the corresponding ADC maps. An abscess collection shows irregular

peripheral enhancement following the administration of an intravenous contrast agent. Gas within the collection may reflect the presence of either recent operative exposure, communication with the skin surface, or extremely rarely, a gas-producing organism. Spinal epidural abscess formation is often associated with adjacent pyogenic spondylodiscitis or infection anywhere along the operative tract. Spinal epidural abscess can cause neurologic symptoms related to spinal cord and/or nerve root compression. Urgent surgical decompression relative to the clinical presentation should be considered in this subset of cases. Nuclear medicine studies may be difficult to interpret in the setting of recent surgical manipulation and implant placement, but, in general, a 3-phase bone scan, indium-111, or gallium scan may show focal uptake of the radionuclide at the site of abscess formation.

In many cases it may be difficult to distinguish an abscess from a seroma or a pseudomeningocele. In these situations, the evaluation and management are driven by the index of clinical suspicion for infection. Blood cultures are often performed and when positive may be helpful. To confirm a diagnosis of suspected abscess, however, image-guided needle aspiration of the fluid collection may be required.[25] This procedure must be balanced against superinfecting a previously sterile collection of fluid. Nevertheless, in an appropriately selected patient with a high index of clinical suspicion, the aspiration biopsy

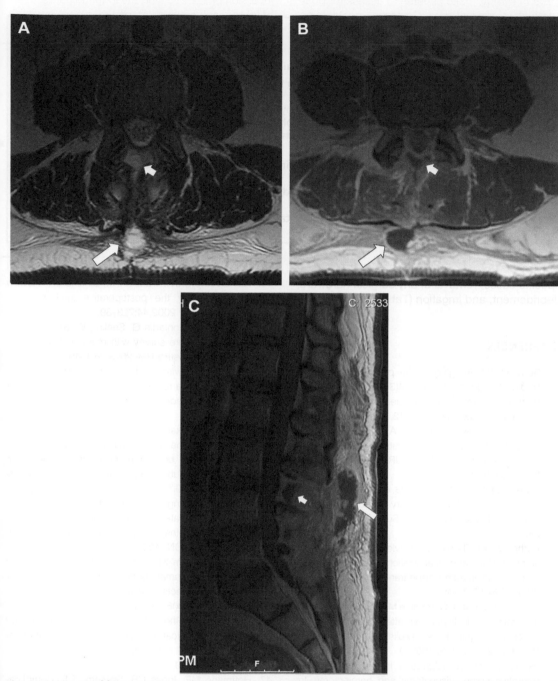

Fig. 9. A 66-year-old man status post L4-5 and L5-S1 laminectomy for lumbar stenosis. T2-weighted axial MR image (*A*) shows a small hyperintense fluid collection (*small arrow*) at the laminectomy site that communicates with a small hyperintense subcutaneous fluid collection (*long arrow*). A contrast-enhanced T1-weighted axial MR image (*B*) shows thick irregular peripheral enhancement about these collections. A midline contrast-enhanced T1-weighted sagittal MR image (*C*) shows complex enhancement with multiple small loculated fluid collections (*arrows*). Subsequent surgical exploration and drainage confirmed the presence of an abscess.

procedure is indicated. Ideally, the procedure should be performed prior to the initiation of antibiotic therapy as the latter will reduce the chances of obtaining a positive culture result. In addition, the

procedure should be performed with strict aseptic technique. The results of the aspiration biopsy will determine subsequent management, which may include antibiotic therapy and drainage or, in

Table 5
Postoperative spine abscess

Definition	A focal circumscribed infected fluid collection
Imaging findings	CT: hypo/isodense fluid collection with irregular peripheral and soft tissue enhancement MR imaging: T1 hypointense, T2 hyperintense, diffusion hyperintense, fluid collection with irregular, prominent peripheral and surrounding soft tissue enhancement. In patients with neurologic deficits, it is important to evaluate for the presence of an epidural abscess
Management	Image-guided aspiration and drainage, preferably prior to the initiation of broad spectrum antibiotic therapy In symptomatic patients with epidural abscess: open surgical drainage and initiation of antibiotic therapy In patients with spinal instrumentation: antibiotic therapy and surgical consideration for revision of instrumentation

specific cases, removal of any surgical hardware, debridement, and irrigation (**Table 5**).[24]

REFERENCES

1. Berquist TH. Imaging of the postoperative spine. Radiol Clin North Am 2006;44(3):407–18.

2. Ross JS. Complications. In: Specialty imaging: postoperative spine. Amirsys; 2012.

3. Hayashi D, Roemer FW, Mian A, et al. Imaging features of postoperative complications after spinal surgery and instrumentation. AJR Am J Roentgenol 2012;199:W123–9.

4. Carreon LY, Puno RM, Lenke LG, et al. Non-neurologic complications following surgery for adolescent idiopathic scoliosis. J Bone Joint Surg Am 2007;89(11): 2427–32.

5. Rutherford EE, Tarplett LJ, Davies EM, et al. Lumbar spine fusion and stabilization: hardware, techniques, and imaging appearances. Radiographics 2007;27(6):1737–49.

6. Kalanithi PS, Patil CG, Boakye M. National complication rates and disposition after posterior lumbar fusion for acquired spondylolisthesis. Spine (Phila Pa 1976) 2009;34(18):1963–9.

7. Van Goethem JW, Salgado R. Imaging of the postoperative spine: discectomy and herniectomy. In: Van Goethem J, van den Hauwe L, Parizel PM, editors. Spinal imaging. New York: Springer; 2007. p. 371–89.

8. Naidich TP, Gologorsky Y, Fatterpekar GM, et al. Complications of surgery for decompression of spinal stenosis and disc disease. In: Naidich TP, Castillo M, Cha S, et al, editors. Imaging of the spine. Philadelphia: Saunders; 2011. p. 513–46.

9. Uribe J, Moza K, Jimenez O, et al. Delayed postoperative spinal epidural hematomas. Spine J 2003;3: 125–9.

10. Van Goethem JW, Parizel PM, Jinkins JR. Review article: MRI of the postoperative lumbar spine. Neuroradiology 2002;44:723–39.

11. Kreppel D, Antoniadis G, Seeling W. Spinal hematoma: a literature survey with meta-analysis of 613 patients. Neurosurg Rev 2003;26:1–49.

12. Sawkar AA, Swischuk LE, Jadhav SP. Morel-Lavallee seroma: a review of two cases in the lumbar region in the adolescent. Emerg Radiol 2011;18: 495–8.

13. Garrett MP, Kakarla UK, Porter RW, et al. Formation of painful seroma and edema after the use of recombinant human bone morphogenetic protein-2 in posterolateral lumbar spine fusions. Neurosurgery 2010;66:1044–9.

14. Benglis D, Wang MY, Levi AD. A comprehensive review of the safety profile of bone morphogenetic protein in spine surgery. Neurosurgery 2008; 62(5 Suppl 2):ONS423–31.

15. Shahlaie K, Kim KD. Occipitocervical fusion using recombinant human bone morphogenetic protein-2: adverse effects due to tissue swelling and seroma. Spine 2008;33:2361–6.

16. Smucker JD, Rhee JM, Singh K, et al. Increased swelling complications associated with off-label usage of rhBMP-2 in the anterior cervical spine. Spine 2006;31:2813–9.

17. Hoffmann MF, Jones CB, Sietsema DL. Complications of rhBMP-2 utilization for posterolateral lumbar fusions requiring reoperation: a single practice, retrospective case series report. Spine J 2013; 13(10):1244–52. http://dx.doi.org/10.1016/j.spinee. 2013.06.022 pii:S1529-9430(13)00697-9.

18. Weng YJ, Cheng CC, Li YY, et al. Management of giant pseudomeningoceles after spinal surgery. BMC Musculoskelet Disord 2010;11:53.

19. Hawk MW, Kim KD. Review of spinal pseudomeningoceles and cerebrospinal fluid fistulas. Neurosurg Focus 2000;9:e5.

20. Ross JS. MR imaging of the postoperative lumbar spine. Magn Reson Imaging Clin N Am 1999;7: 513–24.

21. Thakkar RS, Malloy JP 4th, Thakkar SC, et al. Imaging the postoperative spine. Radiol Clin North Am 2012;50:731–47.

22. Lee KS, Hardy IM. Postlaminectomy lumbar pseudo-meningocele: report of four cases. Neurosurgery 1992;30:111–4.

23. Richards S. Delayed infections following posterior spinal instrumentation for treatment of idiopathic scoliosis. J Bone Joint Surg Am 1995;77-A:524–9.

24. Katonis P, Tzermiadianos M, Papagelopoulos P, et al. Postoperative infections of the thoracic and lumbar spine: a review of 18 cases. Clin Orthop Relat Res 2007;(454):114–99.

25. Diehn FE. Imaging of spine infection. Radiol Clin North Am 2012;50:777–98.

Index

Neuroimag Clin N Am 24 (2014) 391–394
http://dx.doi.org/10.1016/S1052-5149(14)00022-7
1052-5149/14/$ – see front matter © 2014 Elsevier Inc. All rights reserved.

Moving?

Make sure your subscription moves with you!

To notify us of your new address, find your **Clinics Account Number** (located on your mailing label above your name), and contact customer service at:

Email: journalscustomerservice-usa@elsevier.com

800-654-2452 (subscribers in the U.S. & Canada)
314-447-8871 (subscribers outside of the U.S. & Canada)

Fax number: 314-447-8029

**Elsevier Health Sciences Division
Subscription Customer Service
3251 Riverport Lane
Maryland Heights, MO 63043**

*To ensure uninterrupted delivery of your subscription, please notify us at least 4 weeks in advance of move.

Printed and bound by CPI Group (UK) Ltd, Croydon, CR0 4YY

03/10/2024

01040377-0008